HEALTH AND WELLNESS

Journal Workbook

Second Edition

HEALTH AND WELLNESS
Journal Workbook
Second Edition

Brian Luke Seaward, Ph.D.
University of Colorado–Boulder

JONES AND BARTLETT PUBLISHERS
Sudbury, Massachusetts
BOSTON   TORONTO   LONDON   SINGAPORE

World Headquarters
Jones and Bartlett Publishers
40 Tall Pine Drive
Sudbury, MA 01776
978-443-5000
info@jbpub.com
www.jbpub.com

Jones and Bartlett Publishers Canada
2406 Nikanna Road
Mississauga, ON L5C 2W6
CANADA

Jones and Bartlett Publishers International
Barb House, Barb Mews
London W6 7PA
UK

Photographs courtesy of the author. Drawing, p. xvii: Diana D. Tyler's "Three Raptors" used with permission. Copyright © Tyler Publishing, Augusta, Maine. All rights reserved. p. 138, "Muscles of the Soul" reprinted with permission, © 2000, Inspiration Unlimited.

Acquisitions Editor: Kristin L. Ellis
Production Editor: Julie C. Bolduc
Manufacturing Buyer: Amy Bacus
Typesetting: Northeast Compositors, Inc.
Cover Design: Anne Spencer
Printing and Binding: Malloy Lithographing, Inc.

Library of Congress Cataloging-in-Publication Data
CIP data unavailable at time of printing.

ISBN 0-7637-0857-7

Printed in the United States of America
07 06 05 04   10 9 8 7 6 5 4 3 2

This book is dedicated to
Linda Chapin
and the staff of the National Wellness Institute
who have worked so hard and tirelessly
to share the concepts of holistic wellness,
honoring the integration, balance, and harmony
of mind, body, spirit, and emotions.

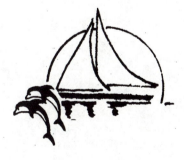

CONTENTS

FOREWORD

A health journal is your personal and private record of your health-related thoughts, feelings, attitudes, perceptions, and behaviors. A health journal allows you to explore your thoughts, attitudes, and behaviors and, perhaps most important, the reasons you behave the way you do at times. When written with honesty, a health journal provides an opportunity for you to stand face to face with the naked truth of your true self. We live in a world where we are always able to work on improving our human potential. This process begins with increased self-awareness. Journaling is considered the best self-awareness tool. Many times the results of journal writing can lead to positive behavioral changes, which is what health and wellness is all about. Students should set aside a few moments every day, perhaps every other day (ideally before or after your health class, if the instructor wishes) to write in your health journal.

Dr. Brian Luke Seaward has provided 76 thought-provoking and soul-searching health and wellness themes that can be used throughout this course. Each exercise provides some background information and then asks you to reflect by responding to specific questions related to each theme. The *Health and Wellness Journal Workbook* integrates all the dimensions of wellness—balancing emotional, social, and spiritual health for total well-being and self-responsibility.

I know you will find this journal workbook to be a powerful tool for learning, self-awareness, and positive behavioral changes that will lead to your highest level of health and well-being.

Kelli McCormack Brown
Department of Community and Family Health
University of South Florida

ACKNOWLEDGMENTS

As the saying goes, it takes a whole village to publish a book, and this book is no exception. First and foremost, I would like to thank all the wonderful people at Jones and Bartlett who share the vision that health is more than just the absence of disease.

Special thanks to Kris Ellis and Julie Bolduc at Jones and Bartlett for making this workbook reach its highest potential.

A heartfelt thanks to my personal assistant, Marlene Yates, whose keen eyes read every word of this book many times over.

Kudos to Kelli McCormack Brown, who as a colleague in the field of health education is a strong advocate of the holistic health philosophy and of my attempt to share this philosophy through my writings.

My gratitude to all those people who use the book as a teaching tool for health promotion.

Thanks to all those people who have dedicated their lives to helping raise consciousness and have served as a tremendous inspiration on my own path; thanks for making this a better world to live in.

And thanks to all my students, who have been wonderful teachers in their own right.

JOURNAL SUMMARY EXCERPTS

The following are some excerpts from journal summaries that I have come across in my several years of teaching college students and journal-writing workshops. These might serve as an inspiration to keep a journal on a regular basis.

The journal helped me to identify what my values are. I found that my values are somewhat different than I had originally thought. I always made the assumption that my beliefs were the same as those of my parents. Although there is some validity to this, there are some areas where my values differ from theirs. Through the use of my journal, I learned how important value definition is in how I perceive things. The last trend that I noticed in my journal was the increasing number and effectiveness of my options for reducing stress. At the beginning, I didn't have any; but as time went on, I came up with better options. I took this to mean that I was learning something—I hope so.

My favorite theme was Unwritten Letters. I thought I had resolved a lot of issues with my former girlfriend, but after having done this assignment, I realized I hadn't. In doing these assignments, I now realize that health is more than just physical exercise. Health begins with a healthy attitude, and my attitude has become much more healthy now that I have gotten to know myself better through these exercises.

For a long time now, I've known what stresses me the most. It has been a long time since I've been able to confide in or let anyone get really close to me. I've been so wrapped up in school for the past eight years of my life, and it's really getting lonely. As time goes on, it gets harder and harder to express myself. In a sense, I'm scared of situations because I don't know how I'll react. In this aspect I don't know myself very well and I'm afraid to find out. This journal has really helped me get in touch with myself.

This stress reduction journal offered no cure-all for my problems, but it gave me valuable help. It helped me understand and see what I thought. By knowing what was going through my mind, I began to realize things about myself, some things I might have never known. A common phrase I saw within my journal was "good enough." The paper was "good enough," the letter I wrote home was "good enough," I was doing things so they would be "good enough," and in doing so, not achieving my potential. I was striving for mediocrity. I'm trying to break this bad habit and I think I have made a little headway. Creativity is now more clear and interesting to me than ever before. I found myself writing short stories in my journal or just creating ideas for work or pleasure.

When I divorced my husband of seven years, I cried on everyone's shoulder for months. That was a year ago. But people get tired of the same old complaints, even your best friends. So I took refuge in writing in my journal. It served as a great sounding board. It certainly helped me heal some very deep wounds. I've learned that there are some thoughts that are better left between my mind and the pages of a journal notebook.

Toxic thoughts! I didn't know I harbored so many of these. I really thought I held an optimistic attitude, but I saw that there is a strong correlation between certain negative attitudes and their corresponding stressors. When the thoughts find their way on paper, they tend to lose their toxic effects in my body. Over the past three months I've seen some things in myself that I often dislike in others. Humm! Very therapeutic. By the way, there were a lot of good times I was reminded of and I'm glad that I have some details to fall back on on occasion. I even found myself in laughing out loud.

Things have always bugged me, but I was never sure what. The journal helped me realize that several things really bugged me and led me to a way to solve my problems. This may sound trivial, but it used to cause me no end of pain. When someone is bothering me and that person asked me "What's wrong?" I always answer, "Nothing." I automatically think they should know what is wrong, but I am wrong in thinking this. I have learned that it bugs me to not tell people they are bothering me. This may seem like a trivial point but I found it a very interesting realization.

Keeping a journal has revealed that I am insecure and unsure about a great many things that I have been putting a false facade on to cover up these feelings. I sometimes think too much, and I often don't think at all. This emotional predicament may cause other people trouble, but I am beginning to take some comfort in my humanness. I look at it this way; someone once said, "Poetry is mass confusion understood." At times my mind is mass confusion. Through my journal if I can begin to understand it, I'll be poetry in action.

JOURNAL THEMES

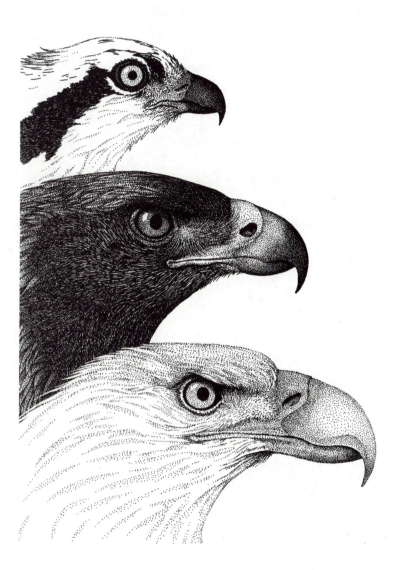

INTRODUCTION TO THE SECOND EDITION

In the six years since *Health and Wellness Journal Workbook* was first published, many changes have happened on the planet. Most recent were the terrorist attacks on the World Trade Center towers and the Pentagon, from which the country is still recovering. No less noteworthy in their own regard are the following: the mass appeal of the World Wide Web; the genetic cloning of Dolly the sheep (as well as the many other animals now cloned); the completion of the Human Genome Project, the entire mapping of the human DNA code; adoption of the euro as the common currency of twelve countries in Europe; scientific agreement on global warming; the last episode of Seinfeld; the first introduction of genetically modified organisms; the first mechanical heart transplant; Americans becoming fatter; and cell phones becoming as common as (but more hazardous than) toothbrushes. Technology has moved from a trot to a gallop, and we humans are trying to keep up with it.

Through it all, life goes on. Students graduate from high school and college. Grandmothers and grandfathers die. Parents retire. Our favorite sitcoms go off the air. New presidents are elected, and the moon turns full every 28 days.

It would be nice if, with all these changes, Americans had gotten healthier, but this appears not to be the case, which is why courses in health education are even more important than ever. By making healthy choices and creating healthy behaviors now, we ensure a better quality of life in the years to come. And given the rapidity of changes on the planet, this can only be a good thing!

Happy Trails,
Brian Luke Seaward, Ph.D.

INTRODUCTION

There is an old mythical story about a young boy who ventures into the forest only to get lost. Completely baffled by his predicament, he wanders aimlessly through the endless miles of trees and brush only to become more frustrated and seemingly more lost. Tired, confused, and hungry, he sits down and begins to cry. Day turns to night and the young teenager curls up to sleep against a tree. The next morning, still crying, he wipes the tears from his eyes to see in front of him an old man holding out a piece of bread. The old man assures the young lad that if he follows the path to the right, he will come upon a stream, which will lead back to his village. Thanking the old man, the boy quickly ventures off in search of home but wanders too far, having been distracted by the sound of rushing water. Eventually the youngster makes it back home, but not without having learned a lesson.

Each one of us is like this youngster—lured by the excitement of the world, but often unprepared for what we encounter. Sometimes reckless in our behavior, we try, at some point, to get back to a level of comfort and security. This journal workbook, like the old man with the piece of bread and directions, is here to provide some guidance and encouragement as you journey on life's path. Just as the old man did not carry the boy back, but rather redirected him, so too does this book serve as a guide, a gentle reminder that while exploration is good, and even encouraged, one must not become too distracted from the path, in this case the path toward optimal health.

To be healthy means to be whole. Wholeness, the premise of wellness, states that the whole is greater than the sum of the parts. What are the parts, the components of the human health paradigm? They are universally accepted as the mental, physical, emotional, and spiritual aspects that comprise a human being. To be healthy means more than just the absence of disease and illness. Wellness means to nurture the integration, balance, and harmony of mind, body, and spirit.

An expression favored by many politicians, clergy, teachers, poets, artists, and executives states "every issue today is a health issue." The reality of this matter came to light in 1993 when efforts were made in the U.S. Congress to pass a health-care reform bill; it failed miserably. Although legislation was blocked, the sad truth is that health problems continue and health-care costs continue to skyrocket. What we do know today is that health and wellness are the cornerstones to virtually everything that we do and come in contact with—the environment, politics, education, religion, the arts, and so much more. We also know that we must take responsibility for our own health—no one is going to do it for us.

When we are young, we tend to take our health for granted. The human body in the late teens and early twenties seems immortal, indestructible, invincible. Even some unhealthy behaviors seem to have minimal effects as the human body rebounds quickly. Unhealthy behaviors, however, have a way of catching up with the finiteness of human tissue and the intricate network of systems that comprise the most dense of human energies—the body.

Journaling has always been insightful and therapeutic. Journal writing can be defined as a series of written passages that document the personal events, thoughts, feelings, memories, and perceptions in the journey of one's life in search of wholeness. Journal writing has proved to be a formidable technique to cope with

3

stress, so much so that psychologists and health educators alike have used journal writing as a tool for self-awareness, self-exploration, and personal development.

The word *journal* comes from the French word *journée*, meaning a day's travel. Journals originated as a means of guidance on long trips, an orientation record for a safe return passage. From Columbus to Lewis and Clark to today's astronauts, journal writing has been and continues to be a means of personal guidance on each individual's journey through life. When pen or pencil is taken in hand and put to paper, a connection is made between the mind and the soul. Putting thoughts on paper makes the writer accountable for those thoughts. The thoughts become real, tangible, and focused; they become concrete. By taking the time to write down the thoughts and feelings that congest or trouble your mind, you develop a habit of clearing your mind of concerns, problems, and issues that constantly demand your attention. Unloading one's thoughts can help clean the conscious mind. It also helps to initiate the process of resolving life's problems. When personal issues are written down, not only is there a cathartic effect, but there is often insight into the stressors, and resolution of these problems begins.

Journal writing opens the doors to your conscious mind and allows you to examine your health behaviors, what you are feeling, where you have traveled in the course of a day, and where this journey has taken you in terms of your mental, emotional, and spiritual growth. By writing in your journal for a period of weeks or months, and later reading through these passages, you will begin to see patterns to your thinking, your emotional responses, and even your actions and behaviors—patterns that are unnoticeable on a day-to-day basis. This is where the real self-learning takes place. From this ability to see patterns in your thoughts and behaviors, you can get a better bearing on how to deal with the issues and concerns that cause stress. Current research suggests that not only is journal writing good for the soul, it is also good for the body. Studies by James Pennebaker, in which individuals kept journals and wrote about their frustrations and painful experiences, revealed that over time they had fewer physical ailments (e.g., headaches, cramps, colds, etc.), which suggests a new bond in the link between mind and body.

The idea for this journal workbook came from a project I assigned to my students as exercises in promoting self-awareness of their health-related behaviors. Generally, I have found that, depending on where each person is in his or her life journey, certain journal themes hold great significance. I have tried to create an assortment of topics, issues, and concerns that I have experienced as well as those I have encountered through the lives of my students, clients, and workshop participants, all of which center on the theme of the integration, balance, and harmony of the mind, body, spirit, and emotions.

At first, journal writing can seem tedious and difficult. This often occurs because we are not in the habit of articulating our innermost feelings. But after a while, as with any skill, you become better at it. Included here are many suggested journal themes to help you get started with the process of journal writing to enhance your self-awareness. These thematic entries motivate and maintain the writing process. They were created to serve as catalysts for soul-searching as well as to give you a jump start when you need motivation to write. You are, however, strongly encouraged to write on your own, with no other theme than "what's on your mind today." There is no particular order to the selected journal themes. You may begin

4

with any theme, or simply write about anything you feel merits your attention. It is important to remember that when you write, write to yourself and for yourself, not to others or for others. The contents of this journal aren't for publication. They are confidential (unless, perhaps, they are assigned for a class or workshop). Your thoughts should be articulated, yet unedited. When you begin to accept this premise, your writing becomes much easier and more honest, and the rewards are more fruitful.

When is the best time to write? This varies from person to person. The end of the day is often ideal, but may not be convenient given your schedule. You really have to decide for yourself. Journal-writing time, however, should be uninterrupted, high-quality, solitary time. How often should you take pen in hand and write? It is suggested that the benefits of journal writing are realized when there is continuity among journal entries. A good initial goal is a minimum of three entries per week. Moreover, journal entries don't always have to be filled with thoughts and descriptions of stressful events based on fear or anger. They can recount good times as well. Life is a combination of positive and negative experiences, and your journal should reflect this. Most important, by keeping a regular habit of journal writing you really begin to know yourself well, and in the process, become your own best friend.

So why a journal about health and wellness? Any health expert will tell you that the first step in changing behaviors is to make people aware of their actions. But actions and behaviors are only the tip of the metaphorical human iceberg. What lies under the water of human behavior are perceptions, attitudes, and values. Until these are explored, pondered, altered, and redirected toward a healthier path of existence, working to change behavior is quite fruitless.

Above all, journaling is an awareness-building technique, to probe the mind and explore your thoughts, attitudes, perceptions, beliefs, and values, as well as your current behaviors. Journaling helps you uncover some of the reasons that you think the way you do; it helps you begin to channel your energies in a way that is more conducive to an optimal path in life.

Within these pages you will find several themes to challenge or support your attitudes, values, and beliefs about your health behaviors. We encourage you to wander through these themes, like the young boy wandered into the forest, and as you do, you will find that the old man who guides you is none other than yourself.

Best Wishes and Inner Peace,
Brian Luke Seaward

I. ACHIEVING WELLNESS

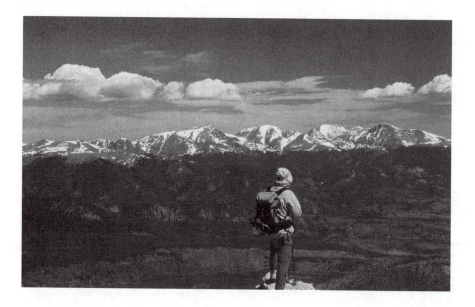

1. MY HEALTH PHILOSOPHY

Life is a kaleidoscope of infinite variety. No two things
are the same. Everyone's life is individual.
Paramahansa Yogananda

We all have philosophies. Philosophies are nothing more than our opinions, dressed up with an introduction and conclusion—a way to present to someone, even ourselves, what we really think about some topic or ideal. We have philosophies on everything—the types of music we like and listen to, the state of world affairs, and even the foods we eat at restaurants.

Now it's time to examine your philosophy about your health. Based on what you already know, and perhaps have been taught or exposed to, as best you can, define what the words *health* and *wellness* mean to you. After having done this, ask yourself why health is so important and write a few lines about this.

Given the premise that every issue is a health issue, identify some seemingly non-health issues like the global economy, deforestation, TV programming. See if you can discover the connection between these issues and the direct link to your state of well-being. Finally, where do you see yourself 25 years from now? If you were to continue your current lifestyle for the next three to four decades, how do you see yourself at that point in the future? Your health philosophy guides your state of health. What is your health philosophy? Be specific. Take some time to write it down here now.

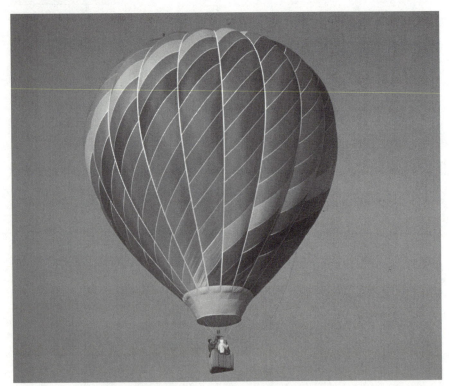

2. THE WELLNESS PARADIGM REVISITED

Ageless wisdom tells us that the whole is greater than the sum of the parts and that all parts must be looked at equally as part of the whole. In terms of health and wellness, the whole is made up of four components: mind, body, spirit, and emotions. Additionally, ageless wisdom suggests that holistic wellness is composed of the integration, balance, and harmony of these four components—that each aspect of our being is so connected to the other three that no separation exists. To look at one component, say our physical health, merits attention to the other three because of the dynamic interconnectedness of the mind, body, spirit, and emotions. What might seem like common sense has not always been so well accepted in the American culture. For over three hundred years, the Western mind has focused on the physical aspects of health, leaving the other three components in the shadows. Since the early sixties the mental, emotional, and spiritual components of health were looked at with somewhat distant interest to the health paradigm; only in the past decade has the interconnection of mind–body–spirit gained respect (and popularity) in Western science.

It has been said recently that every issue is a health issue, meaning that issues such as economic downswings, political instability, rainforest depletion, and moral bankruptcy all ultimately affect our health. To recognize our own health status, we must remind ourselves that we are more than just our physical bodies. We must come to appreciate the true integration, balance, and harmony of mind, body, spirit, and emotions.

Here are some questions to ponder as you explore your own health philosophy, values, and beliefs.

1. Given the dynamics of the wellness paradigm, how does it compare with the common notion that health is the absence of disease?

2. What is your definition of wellness? Do you believe that the whole is greater than the sum of the parts? Can you think of an example in music, politics, or the arts that demonstrates this ageless wisdom?

3. What do you think it means to be an integrated person, to enjoy balance and harmony among your mental, emotional, physical, and spiritual aspects? Do you feel this within yourself? If not, why? Can you identify which aspect(s) you feel are not in balance?

3. TWENTY-FIVE GREAT WAYS TO RELAX

In today's 24-7 lifestyle, taking time to relax is paramount for good health and optimal well-being. There are literally hundreds of ways to relax. A national poll found that the most common is listening to music. Although there is no one-size-fits-all relaxation program, there is a relaxation program that works best for you.

Every relaxation technique works on the premise of deactivating sensory overload that produces an overactive mind. This is done by using one or more of the five senses to reprogram sensory information so that it calms both the body and mind. Because information overload is the result of gathering information through the five senses, it stands to reason that relaxation also involves the five senses, but with a different agenda.

Massage utilizes the sense of touch, music uses the sense of sound, and chocolate employs the sense of taste. You get the idea! Now it's your turn to come up with five ideas on how to relax through each of the five senses. Using the headings for each sense, list five ways to employ that sense to promote a deep sense of relaxation. Be as specific as possible. For example, rather than say listening to music, cite the song or CD, the time of day for listening, and the best location. When you are done making your list, pick one idea from each sense that you haven't done for a long while, or perhaps have never done, and do it this week.

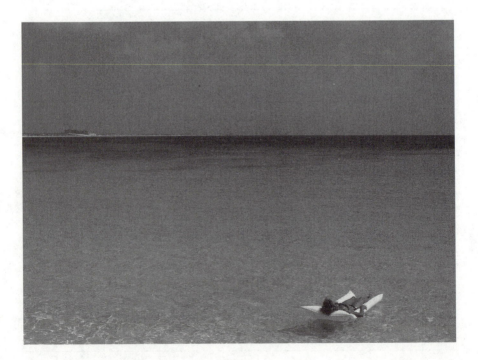

THE ART OF CALM: RELAXATION THROUGH THE FIVE SENSES

List five ideas for each of the five senses, ideas that will help you to relax.

Sight

1.
2.
3.
4.
5.

Sound

1.
2.
3.
4.
5.

Taste

1.
2.
3.
4.
5.

Smell

1.
2.
3.
4.
5.

Touch

1.
2.
3.
4.
5.

4. A GOOD NIGHT'S SLEEP

Sleep is one of the basic human drives. Most health books don't talk much about it, despite the fact that you spend over one-third of your life in that state. The fact is that we tend to take the behavior of sleep for granted, unless of course, we feel we don't get enough of it. The average person sleeps six to eight hours a night, with an occasional nap here and there.

Whatever your sleep patterns were before you came to college, chances are that they have changed dramatically since then. By and large, the freedom connected with college life tends to throw off sleep patterns. Instead of hitting the hay around 10 P.M. or 11 P.M., you might not lay your head on the pillow until 1 A.M. or 2 A.M. On weekends you may go to bed at sunrise, rather than waking up to see it. And let us not forget the all-nighters that tend to become habit forming during midterm and final exams.

Since the 1950s scientists have been studying sleeping behaviors and sleeping patterns in earnest. With over 40 years of data collection you'd think they would have some solid answers; the truth is, no one really knows why we sleep. There are all kinds of theories about the need to have rest, but to date, there seems a lack of evidence as to what actually goes on during the night hours. Interestingly enough, we do know what happens when we don't get enough sleep. Memory and motor coordination fade rapidly and performance, in all aspects, is greatly compromised—as many a college student will attest to when pulling a series of all-nighters.

Describe your sleeping patterns. Are your habits regular? Do you go to bed and get up about the same time every day? How have your sleeping patterns changed since you entered college? Do you make a habit of pulling all-nighters? Do you have problems sleeping at night? Do you have a hard time getting up in the morning? What are some of the patterns you see with your sleep?

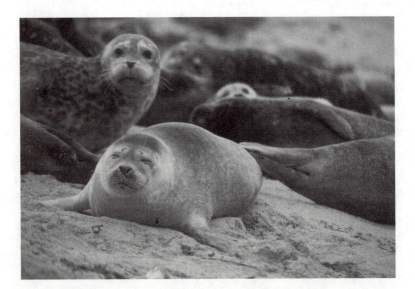

5. EMOTIONAL WELL-BEING

Emotional well-being is best described as "the ability to feel and express the entire range of human emotions, and to control them, not be controlled by them." Sounds like a pretty tall order, huh? Well, it doesn't have to be.

What is the range of human emotions? Everything from anger to love, and all that's in between. No emotion is excluded, meaning it is perfectly all right to feel angry, jealous, giddy, sad, depressed, light-hearted, and silly. All of these feelings comprise the total human experience.

A well-accepted theory suggests that early in our development, we spend the greatest amount of time trying on and exploring emotions. But if you are like most people, you were told at an early age one or more of the following expressions related to your behavior: "Wipe that smile off your face," "Big boys don't cry," "Don't you ever talk back to me," or "I'll give you something to cry about." Perhaps our parents had good intentions, or perhaps they were just at wit's end. Regardless of what prompts such comments, most youngsters interpret the message altogether differently than intended. Instead of relating only to the moment, most children take the meaning of such messages globally and think it is just never OK to laugh or to cry.

If we hear these messages enough, we begin to deny some of our feelings by stuffing them down into our unconscious minds—only to meet them head-on later in life.

The second half of the emotional well-being equation says that to be emotionally well, we must control our feelings, not let them control us. Our feelings do control us when we refuse to feel and express them or when we linger too long in the moods of anger, anxiety, depression, grief, or boredom. The result is stagnation, not dynamic living.

Here are some questions to ponder about your own sense of emotional well-being:

1. What is your least favorite emotion, one that you don't like to feel or perhaps would rather avoid feeling? Can you explain why?

2. Combing back through your memory, can you remember a time (or times) when you were told or reminded not to act or feel a certain way (e.g., big boys don't cry), perhaps even humiliated? Take a moment to describe this incident.

3. What is your favorite emotion? Why? How often would you say you feel this throughout the day?

4. If you feel you may be the kind of person who doesn't acknowledge or express your emotions, can you think of ways to change your behavior and begin to gain a sense of emotional balance?

6. ANCER

He who angers you, conquers you.
Elizabeth Kenny

Anger. The word itself brings to mind images of pounding fists, yelling, and smoke pouring out of one's ears and nose. But anger is as natural a human emotion as love. It is universal among humans. Anger is a survival emotion; it's the fight component of the fight-or-flight response. We use anger to communicate our feelings, from impatience to rage. We employ anger to communicate boundaries and defend values. Studies show that the average person has 14 to 15 episodes of anger a day. They often arise when expectations are not met upon demand. Although to feel angry is within the normal limits of human emotions, it is often mismanaged and misdirected. Unfortunately, we have been socialized to suppress anger. As a result, anger either tears us apart from the inside (ulcers) or promotes intermittent eruptions of verbal or physical violence. In most, if not all, cases we do not deal with our anger appropriately and effectively.

Research has shown that there are four very distinct ways in which people mismanage their anger. The categories include the following types:

1. *Somatizers:* People who never show any signs of anger and internalize their feelings until eventually there is major bodily damage (i.e., ulcers, temporomandibular joint [TMJ] syndrome, colitis, or migraines).

2. *Self-punishers:* People who neither repress their anger nor explode, but rather deny themselves a proper outlet of anger because they feel guilty because they're angry. They punish themselves by eating poorly, neglecting themselves, and so on.

3. *Exploders:* Individuals who erupt like a volcano and spread their tempers like hot lava, destroying anyone and anything in their paths with either verbal or physical abuse.

4. *Underhanders:* Individuals who sabotage or seek revenge through somewhat socially acceptable behavior (e.g., sarcasm, appearing late for meetings).

Although we tend to employ all of these styles at one time or another depending on prevailing circumstances, we tend to rely on one style of mismanaged anger. What is your dominant style? When do situations arise in which you get angry? How do you deal with these feelings of anger?

There are some healthy, even creative, ways to deal with anger. For example, (1) take a time-out from the situation, followed by a time-in to resolve the issue, (2) communicate your feelings diplomatically, (3) learn how to out-think your anger, (4) plan several options to a situation, (5) lower your personal expectations, and most important, (6) learn to forgive—make past anger pass. What are some ways you can vent your anger creatively?

Although anger is an emotion we all experience and should recognize when it arises, it is crucial to manage anger. Sometimes just writing down on paper what gets you frustrated can begin the resolution process. Anger *must* be resolved.

7. FEAR THIS!

We have nothing to fear, but fear itself.
Franklin Delano Roosevelt

Those immortal words spoken during the Great Depression were expressed to calm an unsettled American public. Fear, like anger, is a very normal human emotion. We all experience it—more often than not, too many times in the course of our lives. Fear tends to be a difficult emotion to resolve. Feelings of anxiety or fear can trickle down from the mind to the body and wreak physical havoc from head to toe. While anger tends to make one want to defend turf and fight, fear makes one want to head for the hills and keep on running. The effects of fear can be exhausting. In fact, the effects do exhaust the body to the point of disease, illness, and sometimes death. Avoidance isn't the answer, but it's often the technique used to deal with fear.

Although many situations can promote anxiety, there are really only a handful of basic human fears. They include the following:

1. *Fear of failure:* A loss of self-worth through an event or action that promotes feelings of self-rejection

2. *Fear of rejection:* A loss of self-worth due to a perceived lack of acceptance from someone whose respect is important to you

3. *Fear of the unknown:* A fear based on a lack of confidence or inner faith to act without knowledge of future events or circumstances

4. *Fear of dying:* Anxiety produced by pain, suffering, and uncertainty of death

5. *Fear of isolation:* A fear of loneliness; uncomfortable feelings of solitude

6. *Fear of loss of self-control:* The conflict between the inability to determine factors that are and are not controllable and the feeling of responsibility for total control that produces anxiety

Many of these basic human fears are very closely related and overlap in some instances. Some fears may dominate our way of thinking while others don't relate to our lifestyles. Fear of any kind, however, is very much related to our level of self-esteem. When we are down on ourselves, we are most susceptible to situations or circumstances that we perceive as frightening. Like anger, fears *must* be resolved. Resolution does not include ignoring or avoiding the problem. It is not easy and it takes work. When pursued properly, resolution is a continual process with many fruitful outcomes.

Sometimes by looking at our stressors, we can associate them with specific fears. The following questions may help you reflect on your current stressors that fall into this category.

1. Does one of the basic human fears tend to dominate your list of stressors? If so, why do you suppose that is the case?

2. How do you usually deal with fear? Are you the type of person who hopes the circumstances surrounding these fears will go away?

3. What are some practical ways that will help you deal with some of these major fears?

8. GOOD GRIEF!

If you have ever read the comic strip *Peanuts*, without a doubt you have noticed that Charlie Brown, Lucy, Linus, and Snoopy utter the words "Good Grief." The expression may seem like an oxymoron. How can grief be good? The expression of grief arises from a loss, for example, of a parent, a lover, a spouse, a pet, or anyone or anything of major significance.

Grief is not just a human emotion. It is noted among most, if not all, animals. To feel and express grief is good; when it is not acknowledged and expressed, the residue can have a devastating effect on the body.

The most common sign of grief is the act of crying. Growing up you may have heard "stop crying." A little child interprets that as meaning that crying is not an acceptable behavior. The consequence of this is that we don't learn to grieve properly. In later years our period of grieving can become rather extended, almost in an effort to make up for all the losses we didn't grieve properly as a child. So, the bottom line is that grieving is good. However, there are some caveats. Too brief a time of grieving may be denial of the loss. Excessive or prolonged grieving can lead to depression and thus be a major obstacle on the human journey, preventing you from getting on with your life.

Has there been a time when you were overcome with feelings of grief? What happened? By writing about it, you begin to bring closure to the grieving process, if you are not already there.

Do you ever feel guilty for your feelings of grief? If so, can you trace these guilt feelings to a time or place when your grieving was halted with words like "Big boys don't cry," "Aren't you over that yet?" or something similar to that?

This journal theme invites you to explore your grief, so feel free to add any comments you wish. Good Grief! Go for it!

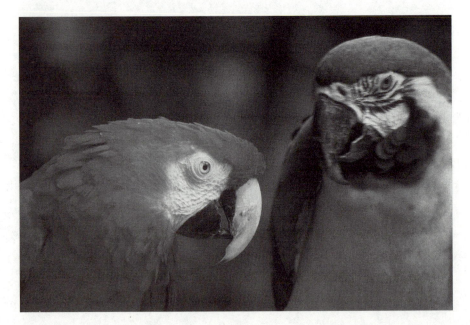

9. ALL YOU NEED IS LOVE

Love means letting go of fear.
Gerald Jampolski

Love. It seems that no other concept has puzzled humankind so much as this. It is love that gives life, and paradoxically, people lose their lives in the name of love. As a professor who studied, taught, and has written several books on the subject, Dr. Leo Buscaglia admits that to define love is virtually impossible. Impossible it may be, but like the elusive Holy Grail, people continue to try. Among authors, poets, songwriters, and actors, the vehicles of love's message are endless.

After years of research, Buscaglia offered his own incomplete definition, suggesting that love is that which brings you back to your real self. In Buscaglia's book entitled *Love*, he writes, "For love and the self are one and the discovery of either is the realization of both." Just as charity is said to begin at home, so too must love reside within the individual before it can be shared. Buscaglia notes that the ability to feel and express love of the self is literally frowned upon as being selfish. In reality, he suggests that to share love you must first give yourself permission to possess and nurture this quality within yourself. Furthermore, self-love begins with self-acceptance, unconditional self-acceptance.

It is interesting to note that the field of psychology has pretty much ignored this emotion during the twentieth century; instead giving the limelight to anxiety and fear. Because of sexual connotations, love as an inner resource has been virtually disregarded, much to the detriment of all human society. More recently, through the works of Buscaglia, Kübler-Ross, Siegel, Borysenko, Moore, and others, this aspect of the human condition is being given more serious attention. In the much-acclaimed book *The Road Less Traveled*, psychiatrist M. Scott Peck offers his insights about love. From empirical observations, Peck perceived that there are many echelons of love: sharing, caring, trust, passion, and compassion, with the highest level of love being a divine essence he calls *grace*.

Let there be no doubt, love is a profound concept. It is a value, an emotion, a virtue, a spiritual essence, an energy; and, to many people, an enigma. Love can inflict emotional pain just as it can heal the scars and bruises of the soul. It can make a fool out of the bravest man and a hero out of an underdog. The expression of love can be quite intimidating as well; and in American society, love is often extended with conditions. Ultimately, such strings taint our perception of love, whereas unconditional love may be the ultimate expression of grace. When people hear the word *love*, visions of Hollywood silver-screen passion come to mind. We have been socialized to think that love has to be as dynamic as Superman, yet the power of love can be as subtle as a smile or a happy thought.

If you were to make an attempt to define love, how would you begin to describe your interpretation of this concept? Is your expression of love limited by your level of self-acceptance? In your expression of love to others, do you find that you attach conditions? In your opinion, how does falling in love differ from unconditional love? Add any thoughts to your definition of love here.

10. IN SEARCH OF THE PROVERBIAL FUNNY BONE

Laughter is the shortest distance between two people.
Victor Borge

Life is full of absurdities, incongruities, and events that tickle our funny bones. For instance, Chaplin once got third place in a Charlie Chaplin look-alike contest. Since the 1964 day that Norman Cousins checked out of a hospital room, into a hotel room across the street, and literally laughed his way back to health from a life-threatening disease, the medical world has stood up and taken notice. Humor really is good medicine.

Today, there is a whole new scientific discipline, psychoneuroimmunology (PNI), to study the relationship between the mind and the body and the effects each has on the other. It is no secret that negative emotions (e.g., anger, fear, guilt, worry, depression, loneliness, etc.) can have a detrimental effect on the body, manifesting as disease and illness. Although there is much to be understood, we now know that, just as negative emotions can have a negative effect on the body, positive emotions (e.g., joy, love, hope, and the feelings associated with humor) can have a positive effect on the body by speeding the healing process and promoting well-being.

Humor is a great stress reducer. Humor acts as a coping mechanism to help us deal with life's hardships. It softens the walls of the ego, makes us feel less defensive, unmasks the truth in a comical way, and often gives us a clearer perspective and focus in our everyday lives. Comic relief is used in many stress management programs, hospitals, and work settings. Stress is often associated with negative attitudes that really deflate self-esteem. A preponderance of negative emotions can taint our view of the world, perpetuating the cycle of stress. There has to be a balance! Researchers are now discovering that we need to incorporate positive emotions to achieve balance, and humor is one of the answers.

Although one can turn on the television to catch a few laughs, the greater variety of humor vehicles (books, movies, live comedians, and music) one is exposed to, the richer the rewards. Sometimes all we have to do is dig through our memory to find a tickler.

1. How would you rate your sense of humor? Do you exercise it often? Do you use it correctly? Offensive humor (sarcasm, racist and sexist humor, practical jokes) can actually promote stress. What are some ways to augment your sense of humor?

2. What is your favorite kind of humor? Parody, slapstick, satire, black humor, nonsense, irony, puns? What type of humor do you fall back on to reduce stress?

3. What would you consider the funniest moment(s) of your life?

4. Are there moments you can recall (from any situation) that are so funny the mere thought puts a grin or secret smile on your face? What are they?

5. In the song "My Favorite Things," Julie Andrews sang about a host of things that flooded her mind with joy and brought a smile to her face. What's on your list?

6. Make a list of things to do, places to go, and people to see to lift your spirits when you need it.

11. VALUES ASSESSMENT AND CLARIFICATION

Values—those abstract ideals that shape our lives. Values are constructs of importance. They give the conscious mind structure. They can also give countries and governments structure. The U.S. Declaration of Independence is all about values, including "life, liberty and the pursuit of happiness." Although values are intangible, often they are symbolized by material objects or possessions, which can make values very real. What are some values? A partial list includes love, peace, privacy, education, freedom, happiness, creativity, fame, integrity, faith, friendship, morals, health, justice, loyalty, honesty, and independence.

Where do values come from? We adopt values at a very early age, unconsciously, from people whom we admire, love, or desire acceptance from—our parents, brothers and sisters, school teachers, and clergy. Values are often categorized into two groups: *Basic values* are a collection of three to five instrumental values that are the cornerstones of our personalities; *supporting* values augment our basic values. Throughout our development we construct a value system, a collection of values that influences our attitudes and behaviors, all of which make up our personality.

As we mature, our value systems also change because we become accountable for the way we think and behave. Like the earth's tectonic plates, our values shift in importance, causing our own earth to quake. These shifts, *value conflicts*, can cause a lot of stress. Classic examples of value conflicts include friendship versus religious faith or social class (Romeo and Juliet), freedom versus responsibility, and work versus leisure (the American Dream). Conflicts in values can be helpful in our maturing process if we work through the conflict to a full resolution. Problems arise when we tend to ignore the conflict and avoid clarifying our value system. The purpose of this journal theme is for you to take an honest look at your value system, assess its current status, and clarify unresolved issues associated with values in conflict. The following are some questions to help you in the process of value assessment and clarification.

1. Make a list of all the values you hold. Values are things that give your life meaning and importance, yet are abstract in nature.

2. See if you can identify which of these values are *basic* or instrumental in your life and which *support* or augment your basic values.

3. How are your values represented in your life? (For example, a BMW may represent wealth or freedom, or the pursuit of an education may be more important than acquiring possessions.)

4. Describe how your values influence your dominant thoughts, attitudes, and beliefs.

5. Do you have any values that compete for priority? If so, what are they and why is there a conflict?

6. What do you see as the best way to begin to resolve this conflict in values? Is it time to change the priority of your values or perhaps discard values that no longer give importance to your life?

12. BRIDGING THE HEMISPHERES OF THOUGHT

In 1956 a researcher named Roger Sperry conducted some experiments on a handful of patients with grand mal epileptic seizures. In the procedure he created, he cut the *corpus callosum*, the bridge of neural fibers that connects the right and left hemispheres of the brain. Not only did the operation reduce the number and intensity of the grand mal seizures, but it also soon gave credence to a whole new concept of how the mind, through the brain, processes information. Roger Sperry's research led to a Nobel Prize in Medicine and to the household expressions *right-brain thinking* and *left-brain thinking*.

Here are some thinking skills allied with the left and right brain, respectively: Left-brain skills are associated with judgment, analysis, mathematical and verbal acuity, linear thought progression, and time consciousness; right-brain functioning is associated with global thinking, holistic thinking, imagination, humor, emotionality, spatial orientation, receptivity, and intuition.

Western culture grooms and rewards left-brain thinking. And it is fair to say that judgmental thinking is one of our predominant traits. While it is true that the Western culture is left-brain dominant in thinking skills, the truth of the matter is that to be dominant in one style of thinking is actually considered lopsided and imbalanced.

1. How would you describe your dominant thinking style? Would you say that your left brain or right brain dominates?

2. If you were to make a guess or assumption as to why your thinking skills gravitate toward one direction or the other, what would be your explanation?

3. One of the basic themes of wellness is balance, in this case, balance of the right-brain and left-brain functions. Based on your answer to the first question, what are your dominant thinking skills and your non-dominant thinking skills? What are some ways you can balance your patterns by bridging between the right and left hemispheres of your brain?

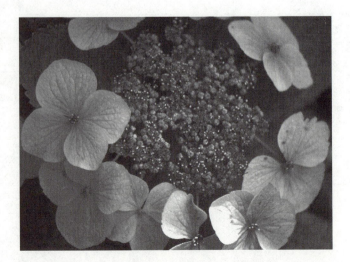

13. MAKING YOUR MARK

Stray not from the path which fate has you assigned.
Ancient Chinese proverb

There are many ways to express our individuality in this world—from the clothes we wear to the style of our hair. But in the long run, how we look doesn't really have an impact on the world we live in. Here is one of the most profound questions you will ever encounter: How will you leave your mark on the history of humanity? The reason this question is so profound is that rather than asking how we will benefit from the world, it asks us how the world will benefit from our endeavors. Making your mark sounds like a shot at immortality, but in reality it is a selfless act of altruism. In the words of President John F. Kennedy, "Ask not what your country can do for you. Ask what you can do for your country."

"Making your mark" is an expression that signifies your positive imprint on humanity. Perhaps a more current symbol is that of footprints. There are many ways to make a mark, a signature expression, yet all of these involve some sense of service, giving of yourself so that others will benefit. Some people volunteer for the Peace Corps, others donate time to local relief efforts, and still others give of themselves in seemingly small but substantial ways to make this a better world in which to live. Music, the arts, and sports are also ways to leave lasting footprints. Above all else, making your mark is nothing less than an act of compassion.

So, how will you make your mark on humanity? This question may seem daunting, but it doesn't have to be. You may already know how you intend to do this. If so, take a moment to share your thoughts and refine your ideas. If this is something you have never given a thought to, now is the time. Start by making a list of your top five interests in life. From there ask yourself what are ways to use your inner resources in these areas of interest so that in some small way you improve the community you live in.

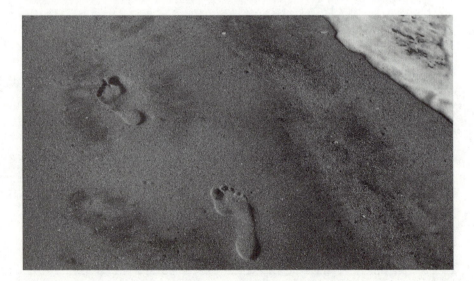

14. THE POWER OF SUGGESTION

Have you ever heard of neurolinguistic programming (NLP)? It is a behavior modification program designed by Richard Bandler and John Grinder based on the concept that words have specific meanings that our unconscious minds pick up on and use to direct our actions, and ultimately, even our state of health (Andreas and Falkner, 1994).

To understand this concept, it helps to know that our conscious mind makes up only a small portion (10 percent) of our total mind. This means that our unconscious mind is really both the navigator and pilot when it comes to behavior. Yet the conscious mind can override the system and cause some problems, especially when thoughts are not congruent with those of the unconscious mind. It gets complicated, but suffice it to say that although the unconscious mind thinks in terms of metaphors and similes, it takes quite literally that which the conscious mind articulates, even when the conscious mind speaks figuratively.

Neurolinguistic programming suggests that the power of words and expressions we use in everyday life can have a big impact on various aspects of our lives. For instance, to say "That sports car is to die for" may carry with it a foreshadowing of a date with the "Grim Reaper." To say that your boss is a pain in the ass may, indeed, foreshadow some lower back pain in the days or weeks to come.

To go one step further, the unconscious mind may suggest a host of expressions that may prophesize the direction of your health, for example, when you say something like "My skin is so sensitive to sunlight that I am a walking tumor waiting to happen."

Neurolinguistic programming invites us to choose our words more cautiously and to get in the practice of thinking before we speak. Remember, the power of suggestion is quite tremendous, especially when the suggestion comes from the depths of your own mind.

1. Take notice of the selection of words you use in everyday conversation. Make note of expressions, idioms, colloquialisms, and vernacular that has both a literal and figurative meaning. List those that come to mind.

2. How often do you use negatives when you speak? If you are like most people, you probably use them quite often. It is said that the unconscious mind doesn't understand negatives. Try converting the negatives to positives. For example, when you say, "I won't flunk this test," the unconscious mind translates this into "I will flunk this test." Jot down all of the negativisms you find yourself thinking or saying and then, next to each, write down a positive expression to use instead. For example, you could say, "I will pass this test."

3. Take note of Freudian slips, or expressions that come out inadvertently when talking. Write these down as well and study them. By and large, they carry a message as well, if we take the time to listen.

15. IMAGINATION AND CREATIVITY

Abraham Maslow, a noted psychologist, studied the positive attributes of human nature. After years of observation, he came to the conclusion that imagination and creativity are the most important aspects of self-actualization, a trait he referred to as that point when we are closest to our divine nature.

As human beings living in a new millennium, we do tend to use our imaginations. But more often than not, we create mountains out of molehills and worst-case scenarios of our problems. If given enough energy and attention, our visions have the potential to become self-fulfilling prophecies.

Let's look at the other side of the coin. We also have the ability to imagine good and positive things. The more detail we can give, the clearer the image and the more likely the ability to bring it into reality. Using the power of your imagination, try writing descriptions of the following themes, giving them as much detail as you can.

1. The best career or job after graduation
2. Your soul mate and life partner
3. Your health forecast for the next decade, year by year

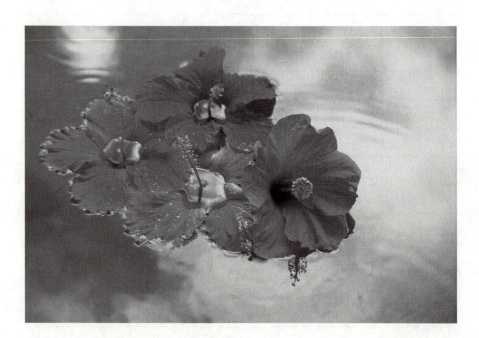

16. BOOSTING YOUR SELF-ESTEEM

No one can make you feel inferior without your consent.
Eleanor Roosevelt

Many themes in this journal workbook revolve around the concept of self-esteem. Self-esteem is considered by many to be the bottom line with regard to the perceptions of stressors and, indeed, how we manage our stress. *Self-esteem* is often defined as our level of self-approval. It is used synonymously with *self-worth, self-respect,* and *self-value.* Ultimately, strong self-esteem equates to the degree of acceptance and love we bestow upon ourselves. High self-esteem can *sometimes* be mistaken and confused with overconfidence, cockiness, and aggressiveness. So, in a humble effort, we tend to compensate. The result is often modesty to the point of negativism, and negativism perpetuates low self-esteem. Today, society gives many mixed messages that *value* both humbleness and greatness. It's a fine line drawn and straddled. We must learn to walk in balance.

Self-esteem is a complex concept. It includes, but is not limited to, acceptance, love, forgiveness, self-understanding, a personal value system, and atonement. Self-esteem is as hard to measure as it is to define. Suffice it to say that at some level each of us knows generally where our self-esteem is, as well as daily fluctuations and things that inflate or deflate it. Most everything we say, think, feel, and do is a function of our self-esteem. In turn, messages that we communicate to ourselves and others from our thoughts, feelings, and actions can reinforce either low or high self-esteem. When our self-esteem is low, we become more susceptible to life's pressures, like a bull's-eye target. Conversely, when we are feeling good about ourselves, problems tend to roll off our backs quite easily. Stress becomes manageable, if even recognized. Four factors contribute to strong self-esteem:

1. *Uniqueness:* Characteristics that make you feel special
2. *Power:* Feelings of self-reliance and self-efficacy
3. *Modeling:* Having a mentor or role model to identify with as a guide on your life journey
4. *Connectedness:* Feelings of bonding and belonging with others, your network of friends and support groups

Take a moment to contemplate the idea of self-esteem, what your threshold is, and the bounds in which it oscillates. What are some ways to increase your threshold for a higher level of self-esteem? Do you see a relationship between your current self-esteem threshold and how well you deal with stress? Try to identify five characteristics that make you unique and give you a sense of empowerment, five role models, and five friends or groups of people you consider part of your support system.

17. LABELS

Every day of our lives we identify things with labels. A red shirt, awful music, expensive books, stupid drivers, or unfair exams. Labels are names we give to various objects that help distinguish them from everything else long enough to get a good handle on them. Labels are impressions we give, through the use of names, to make an association with things. Infants are taught to label things the moment they first learn to speak. The process continues throughout life.

Labels can be nouns, adjectives, and verbs, but mostly they are nouns. Like the strongest adhesive, once we place a label on something, it usually sticks forever. While we may not notice the fact that we label things, people, places, and so on, we surely notice it when we are labeled: fat, stupid, gay, cheapskate, fag, bitch, alcoholic. It's funny to realize that most labels we give to things or other people often outlive their usefulness, particularly labels for people. The reason is that people are not static; they are dynamic. Personalities grow and souls evolve. Labels may be a good beginning of identification, but as good as they may be, they can also limit our growth and human potential. If you are unsure of this, wait till you attend your high school reunion and you will see how much some people really do change.

At best, a label is a form of identification; at worst, it is an acrimonious judgment that can last a lifetime. Let's look at labels from these two perspectives for a moment.

1. How do you use labels to help you navigate the shoals of each day?

2. Do you use labels as a means to judge people? Explain how.

3. Have you found that the labels you have assigned have outlived their usefulness?

4. What labels have been assigned to you by your parents or peers that you not only despise, but know for a fact are not true?

5. What are some ways to successfully and diplomatically erase the unwanted labels you despise?

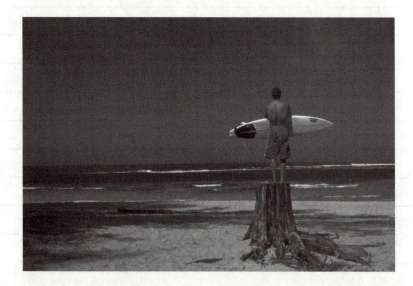

18. MENTAL WELL-BEING

Mental well-being is defined as "The ability to gather, process, recall, and communicate information." If this sounds a bit similar to the way a computer works, there's a good reason. The personal computer is closely based on the functioning processes of the human mind.

There is one aspect of life that can compromise our ability to gather, process, recall, and communicate information. That's stress. Although there are many definitions of stress, one that comes to mind states that stress occurs when we are overwhelmed with sensory stimulation. In essence, our circuits are overloaded. In computer language, the system is down.

Just as the mind needs time to clear itself of thoughts when the circuits are overloaded, the mind also craves stimulation. Mental well-being is that point of balance between stimulation and clarity.

With this definition in mind, what do you do to help clear the mind when you are overwhelmed? (By the way, journal writing is an excellent way to do this.) Learning to cleanse the mind is an essential skill in college because, like no other time in your life, you are constantly being flooded with information to gather, process, recall, and communicate.

Equally important, what do you do to stimulate your mind? As the expression goes, man does not live by bread alone, nor do college students live by lectures, textbooks, and class work. Books for leisure, magazines, the Internet, the Discovery Channel, and museums are just a few ways to seek additional stimulation. What do you do to achieve this balance?

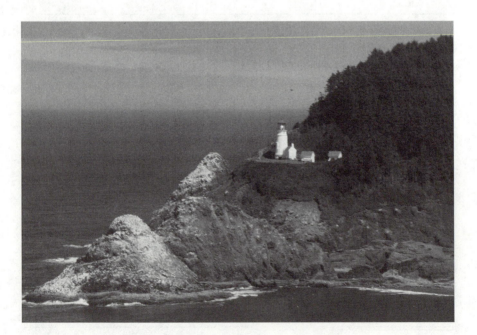

19. WALKING IN BALANCE

*You will have to learn how to balance all of the
Earthwalk's experiences and lessons.*
Jamie Sams
Earth Medicine

A Native American expression describes the concept of living in harmony with nature as always finding yourself "walking in balance." It requires conscious and deliberate effort to achieve balance between mind, body, spirit, and emotions. Knowing that wellness is the integration of these aspects of yourself, what are several ways you can enhance your integration, balance, and harmony? List 25 ideas (activities, attitudinal changes) that can help you walk in balance.

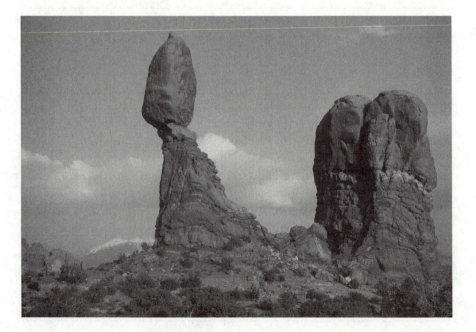

1. _____

2. _____

3. _____

4. _____

5. _____

6. _____

7. _____

8. _____

9. _____

10. _____

11. _____

12. _____

13. _____

14. _____

15. _____

16. _____

17. _____

18. _____

19. _____

20. _____

21. _____

22. _____

23. _____

24. _____

25. _____

20. A BEAUTIFUL MIND

What exactly is intelligence? And perhaps more important, how can we accurately measure it? Would you believe that we don't really know? It's true! It's no secret that there are people with photographic memories who are social buffoons. There are people with excellent street smarts, but it will never show on their GPA. There are those who are great with numbers, demonstrating an impressive fluency with mathematics, yet they appear clueless with all other aspects of life. There are savants who create masterpieces of art but cannot balance their checkbooks. Let's not forget those who are really intuitive. There are also people who see the whole picture of life (and get it), and there are people who are great with minutia, yet who can neither comprehend nor appreciate the big picture. Then, of course, there are the few who are brilliant and seem to have it all together; these people are quite rare indeed.

Intelligence is a funny aspect of being human—funny in Western culture because we think we have a really good handle on what it is and how to cultivate it. Our whole academic system is primarily based on one way of learning. This way is biased toward the capacities and functions of the left half of the brain that favors rational, logical, analytical, judgmental thinking. If the truth be told, there are many ways to learn and there are many ways to assess learning, specifically, right-brain and left-brain functions.

Having said all of this, the question begs to be asked, What is mental well-being? My favorite definition goes like this: Mental well-being is the ability to gather, process, recall, and communicate information. True mental well-being involves a balance of the use of the right and left hemispheres of the brain. It also involves the fluency of thoughts uniting both conscious and unconscious minds. Additionally, it means being both grounded and centered.

In truth, we all have beautiful minds. The real question is, Do we utilize this capacity to our highest potential? OK! It is time to assess your mental capacity and your mental well-being. Here are some questions to help you measure your beautiful mind.

1. Would you consider yourself a right-brain or left-brain person? How would you best quantify your style of intelligence?

2. In terms of mental well-being, which of the aspects (gathering, processing, recalling, and communicating) do you find to be your strongest? Which is your weakest? What ideas can you suggest to improve both strengths and weaknesses?

3. Meditation is a technique used to cleanse the mind. Acts of meditation are similar to cleaning out the old files on your computer before your hard drive crashes. Do you meditate?

4. What activities beside reading do you do to cultivate your intelligence? What creative outlets do you engage in?

5. Here is an interactive assignment. Spend the next 24 hours using your non-dominant hand. This includes writing. Then come back to this page and describe your experience.

21. FIFTEEN MINUTES OF FAME

Most everybody wants to be famous. Why? We all like recognition, and we crave acceptance. Even people who consider themselves introverts like to be considered worthy by their family, friends, and peers. In this age of high technology, the chance of becoming famous is increasing dramatically; it seems like everybody has his or her own television show and web page these days. But fame is never long-lasting. With rare exceptions, fame evaporates quicker than a cup of water in the desert sun. When one face disappears, a new one comes along immediately.

Renowned artist Andy Warhol once said that everybody wants their fifteen minutes of fame. What he meant was that everyone craves acceptance, and many people desire notoriety. Perhaps it's because American culture projects a sense of high esteem for those people who have "made it." When you consider what movie actors and professional athletes get paid compared with what schoolteachers earn, it becomes clear that fame and fortune are American values. Perhaps the real question is, What is success?

The concept of fifteen minutes of fame speaks to more than just the concept of being famous. It really speaks to the concept of ego. Freud is given credit for coining the term *ego*, but in fact the concept of being self-centered is as old as humanity itself. Freud said that the purpose of the ego is to provide pleasure and minimize pain. As bad or big as some egos appear, the truth is, we all need an ego. Our egos serve as our bodyguards. The trouble is that with a great many people, the bodyguard wants a promotion and a new job title (e.g., the boss).

This journal theme is about the topic of ego. Here are some questions to ponder:

1. On a scale of 1 to 10 (with 1 being low), how would you rate the strength of your ego?

2. Do you think egotistical behavior is genetic or a learned behavior? Why?

3. In your opinion, how does ego relate to self-esteem?

4. Do you ever crave acceptance, notoriety, or fame? Why do you suppose this is so? How much of this is influenced by television, magazines, and so on?

5. There is an expression used in Eastern culture: "Domesticate the ego, or you'll have poop all over the place." What are some ways in which you can domesticate your ego and still maintain your self-esteem?

6. Any other comments you wish to share here before you step into the limelight?

22. THE WELLNESS MANDALA

When most people think of health, their thoughts quickly turn to aerobics and broccoli. Perhaps it's all the marketing on television, but in a sound bite, this is what wellness has been reduced to—broccoli and aerobics! Perhaps a little echinacea. As you well know by now, wellness is a lot more than this. Once called the absence of disease, health actually comes from the Anglican word *Hal*, meaning whole or holy. While some people still think of wellness as the opposite of illness, today wellness can best be described as the integration, harmony, and balance of mind, body, spirit, and emotions.

Wholeness, an inherent concept known the world over, is typically symbolized as a circle. The full moon, the Native American medicine wheel, a Christmas wreath, and the Taoist yin-yang symbol are just four of hundreds of examples. A mandala, the universal symbol of wholeness depicted in the accompanying art, is often divided into four parts to signify the four directions (north, south, east, and west). European coats of arms are a derivation of the mandala.

Perhaps by no coincidence, there are also four parts of the wellness paradigm: mind, body, spirit, and emotions, which lends it to the mandala template nicely. Keeping in mind that there really is no separation or division of these four aspects (that's where integration, balance, and harmony come in!), let's use the mandala template to map out your wellness strategy through these four aspects. Using the symbol of the mandala, give some thought to how you foster a sense of wellness, specifically, mental well-being, physical well-being, emotional well-being, and spiritual well-being. Then in each respective quadrant, make a list of what you do to nurture, sustain, and maintain wellness in each of these four areas.

For a variation on this theme, try cutting out a big circle of paper, draw the four quadrants, and then go through the nearest collection of magazines and cut and paste into the quadrants pictures, photos, words, and phrases that apply to each of the four areas. Then hang it up someplace where you can see it every day as a reminder of your highest potential.

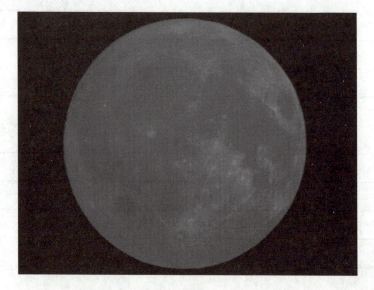

THE WELLNESS MANDALA

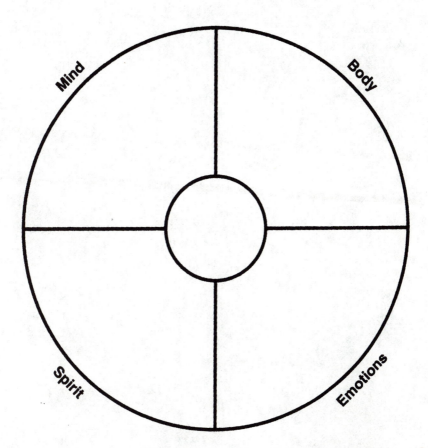

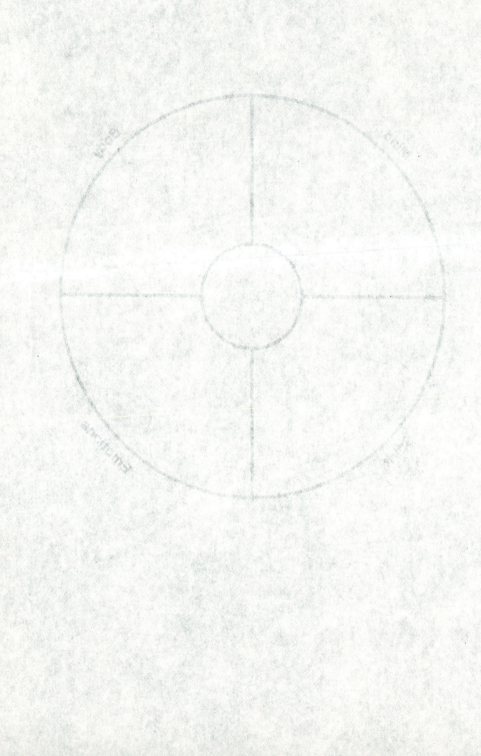

II. A HEALTHY LIFESTYLE

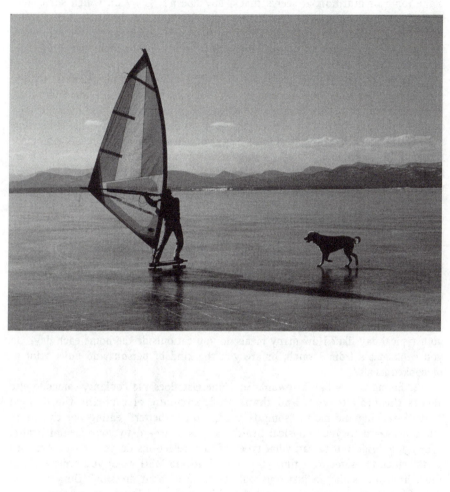

23. FOOD, GLORIOUS FOOD!

If there is one aspect of health and wellness that maintains an air of controversy, it is the topic of nutrition. It seems that a day doesn't go by on which some new scientific study contradicts the findings of a previous study published months earlier. This is good for you, that is bad for you, this causes cancer, that promotes the immune system, and so on. In the search for truth, most people just shrug their shoulders, toss up their arms, and give up.

This we do know: The American diet is top heavy in saturated fats, sugars, salts, and cholesterol. More Americans eat meals prepared outside the home than those cooked at home. These meals are prepared with lots of fats, and hydrogenated oils contain trans-fatty acids that wreak havoc on the integrity of each cell, setting the stage for cancer and heart disease. Fiber content in American diets is extremely low, and this too is thought to be a risk factor for cancer, particularly colon cancer. Let's face it, for a society on the go, the American diet is stopping us dead in our tracks.

You may have heard that the college years are the formative years. This is the chance to explore your freedoms without parental censorship. In terms of food, this means you can eat whatever you want, whenever you want, and you don't have to answer to anyone, except yourself. Everyone knows that college students love food, but as a rule, hate to cook, even if there were time to do so. These factors can set the stage for some pretty unhealthy nutritional habits, which can last a lifetime if they go unaltered.

So let's talk eating habits!

1. Describe your eating habits: How many meals do you eat a day? What is your typical day like? How many meals do you eat outside the home each day? Do you cook meals from scratch, or are you the kind of person who buys a lot of precooked meals?

2. Eating out is like a reward. Someone else does the cooking, someone else serves the food to you, and thank God, someone else cleans the dishes! Notwithstanding the motto "some is good, more is better," eating out can be as much a hazard to your physical health as it is a reward to your mental health. When you do go out to eat, what types of food selections do you make? Are they pretty much the same over time? Do you ask for no MSG when you order Chinese food, limit diet sodas to just one, opt for salad without dressing? Do you avoid deep-fried foods (onion rings, french fries, cheese sticks)? These are just some of the things to be aware of when making healthy eating choices.

3. Do you take vitamin and mineral supplements? If you eat a well-balanced diet, it is probably not necessary. Conventional wisdom, however, suggests that in this day and age no one eats enough well-balanced meals to get what they need in terms of vitamins and minerals. If you do take supplements, are they synthesized or lyophilized? Since the body cannot metabolize synthesized supplements very well, you may be wasting your money. Please describe your habits here.

24. FAST FOOD NATION

*Nobody in America is forced to buy fast food. The first step toward
meaningful change is far the easiest: stop buying it!*
Eric Schlosser

In 2001 Eric Schlosser wrote a landmark book entitled *Fast Food Nation*, in which
he explored behind the scenes of the fast food industry. What began as an article
for *Rolling Stone* evolved into a year-long investigation. What he reveals about the
fast food industry (mostly McDonald's, since they epitomize it) is enough to make
your stomach turn.

Here are some interesting facts from his book:

- In 1970, Americans spent about $6 billion on fast food; in 2000, they spent
  more than $110 billion.
- Americans now spend more money on fast food than on higher education.
- On any given day about 25 percent of the adult population visits a fast food
  restaurant.
- An estimated one of every eight workers in the United States has been
  employed by McDonald's.
- Billions are spent each year to market fast food to toddlers to build life-long
  brand-name loyalty.
- Schools that once housed cafeterias now only carry fast food restaurants.
- Only Santa Claus has higher face recognition than Ronald McDonald among
  fictional characters.
- What we eat (processed foods) has changed more in the last 40 years than in
  the previous 4000.
- The United States has more prison inmates than full-time farmers.
- Every day approximately 200,000 people are sickened by a food-borne disease.
  The most common cause of food-borne outbreaks has been the consumption of
  undercooked ground beef containing *E. coli* 0157:H7 (from animal feces).
- A single animal infected with *E. coli* 0157:H7 can contaminate 32,000 pounds
  of that ground beef.
- A single fast food hamburger now contains meat from dozens or even
  hundreds of different cattle.

More than likely you are among the millions of people who participate in the
daily fast food ritual. Reasons given by most college students include cost and
convenience. It certainly isn't nutrients.

This journal theme asks you to explore your fast food and junk food habits:
What are they, and why do you feel you have these habits? Sometimes by actually
taking time to write down what we do in terms of our behaviors, we begin to see
patterns that we don't normally see day to day. Finally, contemplate this thought.
Schlosser suggests that the fast food industry has had a tremendous impact on
American society as a whole, from poor-quality service to disposable meals. Please
share your comments on this aspect as well.

25. MY BODY, MY PHYSIQUE

Discovering your real self means the difference between
freedom and the compulsions of conformity.
Maxwell Maltz

There is an expression often heard in California that says "Nobody is ever satisfied with their hair." The same could be said about our bodies. We receive hundreds of messages a day from the media telling us that our physiques just aren't good enough! We spend hours and hours and gobs of money altering, complementing, adding, shifting, subtracting, and glamorizing various aspects of our bodies just to please other people in the hopes that we too can be pleased. Hair color, eye color, body weight (too much, too little), aerobic this, anaerobic that, add inches here, take off pounds there; it is fair to say that few people are completely satisfied with their bodies. But it doesn't have to be this way.

There is a strong connection between self-esteem and body image. The two go hand-in-hand. If your level of self-esteem is low, so too will be your body image. In his book *Psycho-Cybernetics*, Maxwell Maltz, M.D., noted that after he performed scores of nose jobs and facelifts, his clients didn't seem all that much happier, which led him to the realization that the real change has to take place inside first.

So how do you feel about your body, your physique?

1. Describe your body. First list all the things you like about your body and explain why. Next, if so inclined, make a list of things you wish to improve.

2. Do you compare yourself to others? If you do, you're not alone. Actually, this is pretty common for both men and women, especially in college when your identity is still being formulated; grooming yourself for that very important first impression can take priority over a term paper every time! So what is it you find yourself comparing with other people? Why?

3. The American public is obsessed with weight and weight gain. There is some good reason for this due to the relationship between obesity and diseases like cancer, diabetes, and heart disease, but the concern has become an obsession for most people. Is your weight a concern for you? If so, how?

4. Taking to heart Maxwell Maltz's notion of making the first change within, can you think of any perceptions, attitudes, and beliefs you can begin to alter so that changes you do make to your physique are long-lasting ones that you feel content with?

26. PHYSICAL EXERCISE

In simplest terms, we are physical animals with a human spirit. As human beings, we were never meant to sit behind a desk for eight to ten hours a day. Human anatomy and physiology were designed to find a balance between motion and stillness, stress and homeostasis, exercise and relaxation. Some would say that the mounting array of disease and illness is a result of being out of physiological balance.

In this day and age, where stress is at an all-time high, our bodies kick out several stress hormones, which if not used for their intended purpose (to mobilize the body's systems for fight or flight) then circulate throughout the body and tend to wreak havoc on various organs and constituents of the immune system. Physical exercise is considered the best way to keep the physiological systems of the body in balance, from stress hormones and adipose tissue to the integrity of bone cells and macrophages of the immune system.

Exercise doesn't have to be all that hard or time consuming. Perhaps more important than what you do is just making the time to do it. Mark Twain once said, "Oh I get the urge to exercise every now and then, but I just lay down till it goes away" (Ayers, 1987). This may be humorous, but the truth of the matter is that physical exercise is what we need to promote the balance and integrity of our physiological systems. Although there is no doubt we seem to have a certain magnetism to the couch and TV, this pattern of behavior has proved to be hazardous to our health.

1. Describe your exercise habits, including the formula for success (intensity, frequency, and duration of exercise).

2. What are your favorite activities? If for some reason you were injured and couldn't do your favorite activity, what would be your second option for exercise?

3. What do you do to motivate yourself when you are less than inspired to get up and out the door? What are some additional incentives to maintain a regular exercise regimen?

4. Most people say that they cannot find the time to exercise. Considering classes, studying, work, social obligations, and the like, it is hard to fit in everything. So the question of priorities comes to mind. What are your priorities in terms of your health? Do you see your perspective changing in the course of your life? Right now, what can you do to find (make) the time to get physical exercise every day?

5. Sketch out a quick weekly program of exercise, including days to work out, time of day, and activity.

27. FRANKENFOODS

Let food be your medicine and medicine be your food.
Hypocrites, father of Western medicine

What is your relationship with food? Do you buy your food frozen, prepackaged, freeze-dried, or canned? Do you cook your own food or does someone typically do it for you? It is interesting to note that Americans are up in arms about human cloning, yet no one seems to even notice that scientists are splicing the DNA of flounder into tomatoes, the genes of rats into hogs, and the pesticide Roundup into the DNA of corn. The Kellogg Company had to recall millions of boxes of Corn Flakes in 2000, and Taco Bell recalled thousands of taco shells because of the hazards of genetically modified foods. Those people who are allergic to peanuts now have to watch the corn products they eat. Cross-species gene splicing has made corn a dangerous food to consume. In fact, many food allergies are thought to be related to genetically modified organisms (GMOs).

Food experts suggest that as many as 70 percent of the produce and processed foods in the grocery store are genetically modified. At the top of the list are tomatoes (which includes ketchup, tomato sauce, and salsa), corn, and soy. By the time you read this there could be many, many more. Effective lobby efforts in Congress by the Monsanto Corporation have allowed these foods to go unlabeled.

1. What types of foods do you buy in the grocery store?

2. What percentage of meals do you eat outside the home each week?

3. What percentage of foods do you buy that are organic?

4. Are you allergic to any foods? If so, which ones? Have you noticed being allergic to more foods in the past five years than before this time when GMOs were introduced?

5. Go online to your favorite search engine and type in the words *Frankenfoods* or *GMO*. Check out three or four websites and write down some of the highlights you find.

6. After you have done this, take a few minutes to write down your thoughts on the topic of Frankenfoods.

28. IS FAT REALLY WHERE IT'S AT?

Transfatty acids are so unnatural, even bacteria won't go near them!
Doug Margel, D.O.

Perhaps you have heard—America has a weight problem! Over 50 percent of Americans are considered obese by several standards, including body composition tests and body mass index (BMI). Although there are several factors related to obesity, one of the first to address is the types of foods that we eat. Much attention has been placed on saturated fat and cholesterol, but this is only the tip of the iceberg, if not the food guide pyramid.

In the early twentieth century, scientists began to experiment with lipids to reduce the rate of rancidity. In essence they were looking for ways to prolong the shelf life of processed foods that contained fat. Their legacy has haunted us ever since. It is virtually impossible to find any packaged food without "partially hydrogenated oil" listed in the ingredients. Examples include everything from cookies and potato chips to cereal, pancake mix, and peanut butter. Hydrogenation of oils (making a lipid a saturated fat at room temperature) created transfatty acids. Current research suggests that these act like free radicals. In essence, they destroy the integrity of various cells, including the cell wall, DNA, RNA, and mitochondria. Transfatty acids are linked to both coronary heart disease and cancer. And they are most definitely linked to the obesity problem in America. Why? Because these types of fats are not natural, and once absorbed into the body, the body has no idea what to do with them. In small amounts they may not appear to do much, but over time they can cause a real problem.

Here is your assignment: Go into your kitchen and open the cupboards and refrigerator. Start looking at the list of ingredients of the foods you find and make a list. Most likely you will be amazed at what you find.

Here is another problem! Your body has to have omega-3's (cod fish oils and flaxseed oil) and omega-6's (vegetable oils). But nowhere on the food guide pyramid does it say you have to have these. These are called essential fatty acids because your body cannot make them—they have to be consumed from the foods you eat. The problem is that in our fat-phobic society, people are not getting the correct balance of essential fatty acids (not enough 3's and too much of 6's). A lack of essential fatty acids is now thought to be a determining factor in several chronic diseases. Are you getting enough of these? Are you getting the right balance? Go back into the kitchen and see if these sources of oil are in your fridge and come back and report what you find.

29. THE SEROTONIN BLUES

It's hard to believe that in a country as great as the United States, where the living standard is the envy of almost every other nation in the world, about one-third of the population is diagnosed with or being medically treated for depression. Something is terribly wrong with this picture! In a land where the American dream states that "You can have it all," this promise certainly has its drawbacks.

Medical scientists have known for several decades that at the biochemical level, depression is related to a decrease in the hormone serotonin, a special neurotransmitter that regulates a great many physiological processes in the body. The relationship between and among neurotransmitters in the brain is complex, to say the least. Serotonin works in conjunction with dopamine and melatonin as well as several other neuropeptides. These in turn also seem to have a great effect on our emotions.

The biomedical model of well-being is myopic. It only sees brain chemistry having an effect on emotions, not the other way around. The biochemical model also falls short of recognizing that many of the foods we eat play a significant role in brain neurochemistry. These include a host of artificial flavors, colors, preservatives, and sweeteners.

Freud once said that depression is anger turned inward. Indeed, depression is more complex than the levels of serotonin produced in the brain. But this is a good place to start to look and see how we might be affected.

Most likely there is a good chance that you or someone you know has been depressed. This journal theme is dedicated to the topic of depression. It offers you a chance to write about how you feel when you become emotionally overwhelmed. Thinking holistically, what steps can you take to move out of the shadow of depression though mind, body, spirit, and emotions?

30. FOCUS!

Are you one of the millions of Americans diagnosed as having ADD, someone with an attention deficit disorder? If you are, you are in good company. It seems nearly everyone has a shortened attention span these days. It may be hard to imagine, but not long ago, television commercials were 30 to 60 seconds long. Then came the invention of the remote control. Now commercial sponsors duel with your attention span in the hopes they can get their message across before your thumb makes a move. Add to the equation the introduction of video games and it would appear that technology has played a very big role in undermining the national attention span. But that is not all. There are a host of chemical substances we ingest, often without knowing, that also affect our conscious thought process.

In his book *Excitorins*, author Raymond Blaylock describes various food substances that greatly affect brain function. The two most commonly ingested excitoxins include aspartame (more commonly known as Nutrasweet and Equal) and MSG (monosodium glutamate). These two substances, as well as a host of artificial colors, flavors, and preservatives, have a serious effect on cognitive function. Aspartame and MSG cross the blood-brain barrier.

More than likely the ability to focus your attention is based on the coming together of a great many factors. Here is a chance to look at your health behaviors and see if there are things you do that contribute to a poor attention span. Here is a challenge: Come up with ten behaviors you partake in that you feel decrease your mental focus. Explain each one.

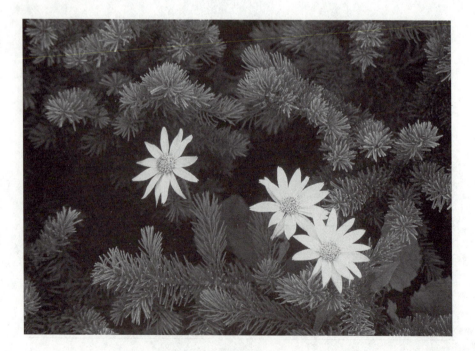

1.

2.

3.

4.

5.

6.

7.

8.

9.

10.

III. HEALTHY RELATIONSHIPS

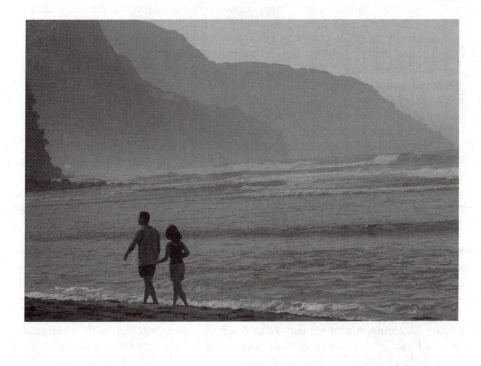

31. SEXUAL INTIMACY

Sigmund Freud is credited with having said that the average adult thinks about sex every 30 seconds. While the time interval may vary from person to person, there's no doubt that our sexual drive, along with our drive for nourishment and sleep, is an important part of our daily makeup. Consequently, sexual drive can contribute to frustration and stress. Regardless of gender, individuals become sexually aware (and perhaps active) during puberty, around the ages of 9 to 15 years. Not until a person reaches adulthood (said to usually be at about 18 years) is his or her sexual behavior fully recognized and accepted. Between puberty and adulthood there exists a 3- to 9-year period of potential personal frustration.

Social, cultural, and religious mores and expectations may confound the issue with rules, laws, and dogma linking the approval of sexual activity with marriage. What can be really confusing are all the mixed messages from the media and advertising industry that are loaded with sexual overtones and innuendoes linking sexual activity with beauty, success, popularity, and so on. Moreover, there are many issues and concerns adding to the confusion, including unplanned pregnancy, sexually transmitted diseases, rejection, birth control, values conflicts, rape, homosexuality, and guilt. Later in life, more issues arise that are related to sexual anxiety, including not being able to conceive, low sperm count, sexual addiction, impotence, sexual inactivity, and sexual dissatisfaction.

Unlike our other drives, human sexuality carries the heavy burden of incredible responsibility. As a result, the issues surrounding sexuality can be very stressful. Without a doubt, good communication is a crucial factor in reducing some of the anxiety regarding human sexuality. The communication must start with ourselves, to ourselves, and from there to those with whom we are intimately involved. Now is a good time to initiate this communication with yourself. Is sexuality a current stressor in your life? Please take a moment to do some soul-searching on this issue.

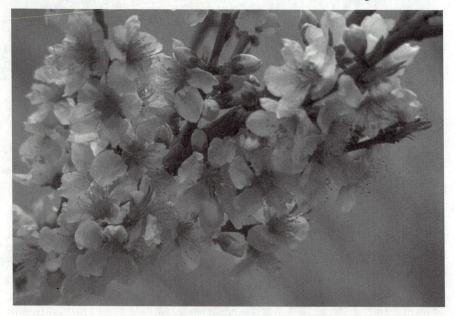

32. THE STORK HAS ARRIVED!

Pregnancy and parenthood bring on the entire spectrum of human emotions.

Dan H.

There is an expression that notes there is no such thing as being a little pregnant. You either are or you are not. The reaction to the discovery of pregnancy is much the same way. You are either delighted or you are not. Given all the factors involved with being pregnant or getting your partner pregnant, your emotions can run the gamut. A friend called me the other day to tell me the news that his girlfriend was now pregnant. His response ran up and down the emotional spectrum. He was happy and nervous in the same breath. Not being married was a factor, as was the issue of fatherhood. There is a funny irony to pregnancy. In the teen years this condition is something to avoid like the plague, yet once married, there seems to be a lot of effort to achieve pregnancy, with disappointed expectations. As the saying goes, "there is no such thing as an unplanned pregnancy."

If you find yourself in a serious relationship, this is a matter to give some serious thought to. How would you feel discovering that you are pregnant (women), or that you have impregnated your partner (men)? What emotions surface just thinking about this prospect? Why do you feel this way? If you were about to become a parent, what things would you plan to do so that you would or would not act like your parents? What are some rules and boundaries you wish to establish to break any negative cycles from your family history? Take some time to write about your thoughts and feelings. Taking the time to do this now will make it all the easier to process these feelings when the day comes that indeed the stork arrives.

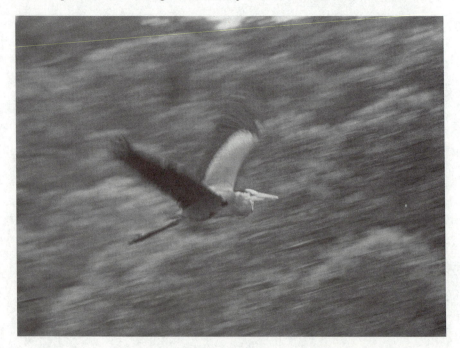

33. WHAT DID YOU SAY?

Conversational skills may not seem like they belong in a health and wellness book, but nothing could be further from the truth. We are engaged in conversation from the moment we wake until the second we lay down our heads and enter the world of dreams. Whether it be family, friends, customers, clients, peers, colleagues, strangers, or even voices on the radio and television, our minds are programmed to listen and respond in conversation virtually every minute of the day.

An old proverb states "The three most important words to a successful relationship are communication, communication, communication." It's true! As social animals we gravitate toward others to engage in conversation. Good communication skills are essential to every aspect of our lives. The elements of conversation are rather complicated because we communicate with more than just words and voices. In fact, more of our communication skills are nonverbal than verbal.

1. How good are your communication skills, both verbal and nonverbal? Are you even aware of the messages you give to others with your clothing style, your hair, eye movements, posture, hand gestures, and facial expressions?

2. What would you say is your body's silent message, that is, without dialogue? Why? Is this the message you wish to convey?

3. Listening skills are as important as the ability to articulate your thoughts and feelings. Yet, most people hear, but seldom listen. More often than not, they begin to prepare what they are going to say within seconds of someone's beginning to speak or respond. How good are your listening skills? What could you do to improve them?

4. Much research now suggests that men and women have different styles of communication. Have you ever noticed this? For example, have you noticed that when a woman says she'll call you tomorrow, she calls you tomorrow, whereas when a man says he'll call you tomorrow, most likely he will call you in a few days to a week?

5. It has been said that when we speak we are very indirect, not really saying what we mean. We beat around the bush. Do you find your verbal style is more indirect than direct? Do you tend to give mixed messages? After giving this some thought, can you think of ways to improve your verbal communication skills? Do you need to revise your nonverbal messages? How can you do this?

6. Men and women are said to have different communication styles. While it may be true that men are from Mars and women are from Venus, we are both here on earth, so we have to learn to be bilingual. What differences do you notice talking to the opposite gender? How are these differences magnified in a relationship? Share your thoughts and experiences here.

34. TAKING A STAND ON BIRTH CONTROL

Human sexuality is a normal and healthy component of our well-being. Yet, a quick look at the notion of sexuality is confusing at best. The American culture is often noted for sending incredibly mixed messages regarding sexual behavior. The media thrives on using sexuality to sell products (e.g., jeans, cars, vacations, perfumes). Several religions cast blame and guilt as a means to control sexual behavior.

If you engage in sexual activity, undoubtedly you will come face to face with the issues of birth control, abortion, and sexually transmitted diseases, including AIDS. The time to form an opinion about these issues is not after you have engaged in sex, and are then forced to make a decision because of a consequence. The time to form an opinion is before you act. You should feel comfortable enough to stand by your opinion until you feel moved to rethink and reformulate it. Ask yourself this now: What is my stand on issues like birth control, abortion, and the exposure to AIDS? Has it always been this way? Is my opinion based on accurate information, on my own experience, on my parents' beliefs, on media messages, on peer pressure? Any other comments you wish to add here?

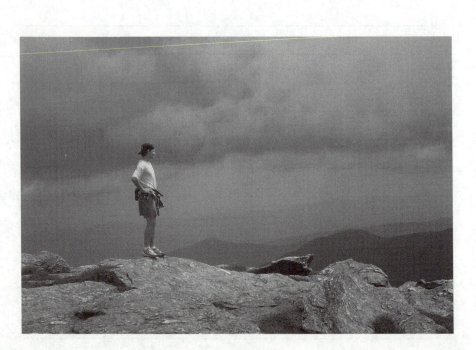

35. UNWRITTEN LETTERS

Many times we want to say something to someone we love, like, or just know well. For one reason or another, whether it be anger, procrastination, or not finding the right words at the right time, we part ways. As a result, those special feelings never seem to be resolved. There was once a college student whose former boyfriend took his life. In the note left behind, he specifically mentioned this student and his words haunted her for what seemed like an eternity. Through some counseling, she decided to write him a letter to express her anger, sorrow, loneliness, and love. Her words, her letter, began the resolution process and her path toward inner peace.

Resolution through letter writing has been the theme of a great many books, plays, and movies. In a movie made for television, *Message to My Daughter*, a young mother with a newborn baby discovers she has terminal cancer. As a part of her resolution process, she records on several cassette tapes personal messages to her daughter. Many father–son relationships also fall into this category, where men feel that their sons might never get to know them in their own lifetime. It is a common theme found in movies, plays, and books because, as the expression goes, "Art imitates life."

Perhaps because of the recent advances in technology, from the cellular telephone to the microchip, Americans are writing fewer and fewer personal letters. Sociologists worry that future generations will look back at this time period, the high-tech age, and never know what individuals were actually feeling and thinking because there will be few written records. Moreover, psychologists agree that many of today's patients are troubled and unable to articulate their thoughts and feelings, thereby resulting in unresolved stress.

This journal entry revolves around the theme of resolution. The following are some suggestions that might inspire you to draft a letter to someone you have been meaning to write. Now is your chance.

1. Compose a letter to someone you were close to who has passed away, or perhaps someone with whom you have lost contact for a long period of time. Tell that person what you have been up to, perhaps any major changes in your life, or changes that you foresee in the months or years ahead. If there are unresolved feelings toward this person, try expressing your thoughts and feelings in appropriately crafted words so that you can resolve them and come to a lasting sense of peace.

2. Write a letter to yourself. Imagine you have one month to live. What would you do in these last thirty days? Assume that there are no limitations. Whom would you see? Where would you visit? What would you do? Why?

3. Pretend that you have a baby son or daughter. What would you like to share with your child now, in case, for some reason, you do not have the opportunity to do so later? What would you like your child to know about you? For example, perhaps you would share things that you wanted to know about your parents or grandparents that now are missing pieces of your life.

4. Write a letter to anyone you wish for whatever reason.

36. THE MALE ENIGMA

If a man speaks in the forest and there is no
woman to hear him, is he still wrong?
Anonymous

Let's face it, guys, it's not easy being male these days! There are hundreds of messages saying to be manly and macho, while at the same time there are messages to be sensitive and understanding. What's a guy to do? The last thing you want to do is reveal too much about your inner self so as to look vulnerable by showing your feelings to other guys, but this is what women really want to see. So being male either means being a great actor or walking through life with a poker face. Either way, this persona invites problems.

There was a time when a man's role in life was fairly well established. The man of the house was the provider, the breadwinner, and the one who cooked meals on the barbecue. The woman raised the kids, cooked the rest of the meals, and kept house. Then came the feminist movement and all the rules changed. Now women have more freedom in career choice, but no one cooks, they just order out, and daycare professionals raise the kids. The sad news is that after over 30 years of female liberation, the male life expectancy is still 5 to 10 years less than that of women, and these days everybody's on Prozac or Zoloft. Go figure!

Somewhere between machismo and New Age sensitivity there has to be a balance. Here is how one guy put it: "I realize that I care about others' feelings more than I let on. I think that I have more of a sensitive side than most guys would admit to, but this is by no means a bad thing. I looked at my values, which is something that I hadn't done in a long while, and realized I needed to focus more on the values that I was raised with than the values of my friends. I also realize that I have a great distaste for violence against another human being. I strongly believe that violence is a way for people who don't know how to deal with their feelings properly to relieve themselves of this perceived negative."

This theme is just for the guys (sorry, ladies!). Here are some questions to ponder and then express yourself about.

1. What is it about being a guy that you like?

2. What is it, if anything, about being a guy that frustrates you?

3. Why do you think it is hard for guys to express their emotions to other guys? Do you ever do this?

4. If machismo is on one side of the scale and sensitivity is on the other, where do you see yourself and why? Is this something you model from your father or some other male role model, or is it something you adopted on your own? Please explain.

37. FRIENDS IN NEED

And let there be no purpose in friendship, save the deepening of the spirit.
Kahlil Gibran
The Prophet

What is a friend? Perhaps it's someone with whom to share precious moments of your life. Perhaps a friend is a person to whom we confide our innermost thoughts and feelings. Maybe a friend is someone just to be there when we need a helping hand or a comforting hug. Friends are all this and more.

Human beings are social by nature. Although times of being alone can serve as a great way to energize the soul, it is to our advantage to balance solitude with interactions. We need exchanges with people to whom we feel close, our network of friends and family.

Some interesting findings have emerged from research investigating the health and longevity of the world's oldest living citizens. We now know that involvement with friends, who make up our social support group, are as important to our health as regular exercise, proper nutrition, and sleep. It seems that in troubled times our friends can help buffer or neutralize the stress and tension we feel and serve as an effective means to cope with stress.

As we grow and mature in our own lives, so do the relationships with our friends. The bonds we have with some people continually strengthen over time and distance while others seem to fray or fade. We often attract people into our lives with similar interests and ambitions. In some cases, our closest friends can seem more like family than our brothers and sisters. In every case, friendships, like house plants and pets, need attention and nurturing. Every now and then, it is a good idea to take a moment to evaluate our friendships, to see if they are truly fulfilling our needs. This inventory of friends can let us know if we have outgrown, or grown apart from, some people, and why. It can also make us aware of the qualities that comprise a good, close, or best friend, and the difference between a good friend and an acquaintance. We also need to evaluate if we are making an equal contribution to each relationship. Here are some questions to help you with this assessment.

1. How would you best define the word *friend?* What does being a friend mean to you?

2. What is it that draws a person into your life to become a friend?

3. Make a list of all your current friends. Are any members of your family in this group? How has this list changed over the past five years?

4. How would you evaluate your current circle of friends? Do you have several acquaintances that you call friends?

5. Does your support group consist of people in different social circles, or is yours a closed circle of friends? Why would friends in different circles be of value?

6. What keeps your bonds of friendship strong and what tends to let some friendships fade away?

7. Are there any additional comments you wish to add here?

38. SIX DEGREES OF SEPARATION

Do unto others as you would have them do unto you.
The Golden Rule

Conventional wisdom suggests that we are all connected at some level. Physicists agree that at some level we all share the same molecules. Moreover, some people say that if we look at our genetic lines, we will find that we are a lot more related than meets the eye. Some estimates suggest that everyone is "at least a cousin, 16 times removed."

A common way to emphasize our connectedness is the expression "six degrees of separation." What this originally meant was that we are six people away from knowing someone famous. There was even a game created on this theme called "Six Degrees of Kevin Bacon." What this suggests is that we are six people away from knowing just about everybody on the planet. Some say this is an exaggeration, while others say there are no degrees of separation.

If you stopped to map it out, you are probably six or fewer people away from knowing the following people: Lance Armstrong, Bill Clinton, Jewel, Michael Eisner, or Julia Roberts. This gives a lot of credence to the expression "It's not what you know, but who you know that counts." Most likely it is a combination of both, but the fact remains that connections count. With the events of September 11, the degrees of freedom were reduced from six to two, or so it seemed. Everyone seemed to know someone who was either directly or indirectly affected by this tragedy.

This theme invites you to reflect on the topic of relationships. Make a list of ten people in your life whom you consider to be your best and closest friends. Compare this list to the list of people whom you would have placed on it ten years ago. Are any of the people on both lists? What does it mean to be a friend and what do you do to cultivate these relationships? How do your friends contribute to your overall sense of well-being?

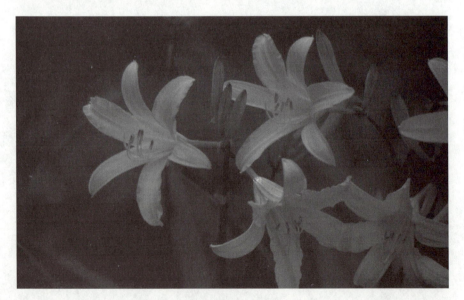

39. REINVENTING YOURSELF (AGAIN)

We enter this world with a clean slate, yet from the first day, our behaviors and mishaps and, later, our accomplishments (or lack thereof) begin to define who we are to everyone we meet and know. Through our thoughts, words, and actions we paint a composite that we present to the world. As we mature from teenagers to adults, many of the things we did in our early years serve as a constant reminder of the mistakes or poor judgments made along the way. And there are always people (such as our parents) who remember us as we were, not as we have become.

Going to college provides a great means to wipe the slate clean again and start anew. New people, new friends, and new relationships lay the foundation for a refined image of who we are evolving into. Reinventing yourself is best described as taking your best qualities and building on them. Reinventing yourself is not running away from all your troubles and worries and pretending to be someone you are not. Instead, reinventing yourself is maturing your finest qualities and leaving behind those aspects that don't serve your highest good. Of course, it really helps when you can do this in a new environment where the slate is truly clean.

Here is the catch to reinventing yourself. You have to start from the ground up. This means that you have to know in your mind how you want to be, how you want to act. Reinventing yourself begins in the mind long before it manifests itself in your actions.

Why would you want to reinvent yourself? Simple! Perhaps you have been attracting the wrong kind of person in your intimate relationships. Perhaps you keep finding yourself in the same kind of meaningless job. There are many reasons.

So if you were in the frame of mind to reinvent yourself, where would you start? Attitude, food, clothes, movies, music, haircut, or all of the above? Knowing that reinventing yourself begins in the mind, consider that your slate is now clean. Make a list of ten things you can do to create the new and improved you.

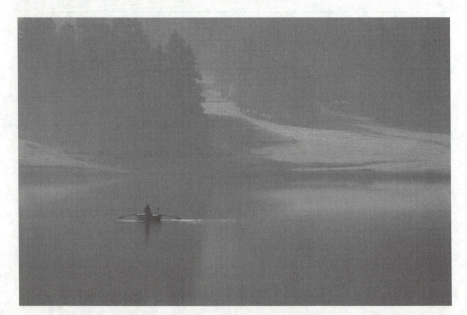

IV. PREVENTING DISEASE

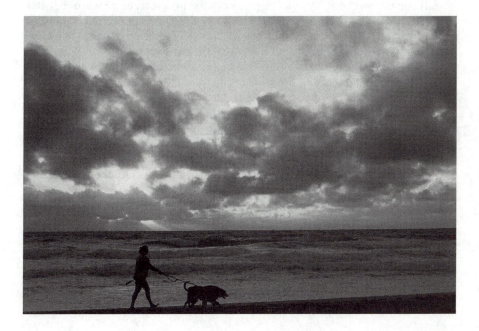

40. MY HEALTH PROFILE

Health is so much more than the optimal functioning of our physical bodies. But when it comes down to it, by and large, this is what people focus on when they talk about health. To fully understand the mind–body–spirit connection, you must realize that the body is actually the endpoint where unresolved issues of mind and spirit collect, not the beginning. But *if* we were to start with the body and examine, from head to toe, our physical makeup, perhaps we could use this as a stepping-stone to understanding this unique relationship.

Several aspects of our physical makeup, when looked at in a composite, tend to give us a sound understanding of our physical health status. This journal theme invites you to take some time to explore your overall physical health. Once you have compiled all your personal health data, compare your values with the norms discussed in class, or in the book *Health and Wellness*. If you should have any questions regarding your profile, bring these to the attention of your physician.

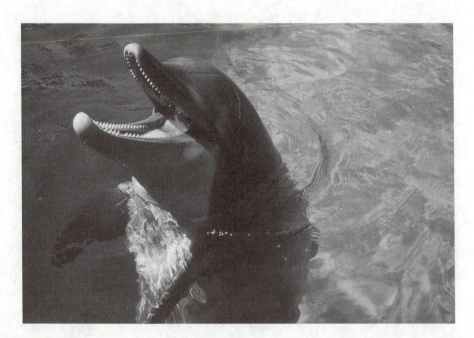

MY HEALTH PROFILE

Name _____

Height _____

Weight _____

Age _____

Resting heart rate _____

Target heart rate _____

Maximal heart rate _____

Resting systolic blood pressure _____

Resting diastolic blood pressure _____

Total cholesterol _____

HDL level _____

LDL level _____

Vision status _____

Dental status _____

Hearing status _____

Skin condition _____

Gastrointestinal tract _____

Tense areas, muscular _____

Reproductive system _____

Skin _____

Sinuses _____

Other _____

_____

_____

_____

41. CLIMBING THE FAMILY TREE

By the time you read this sentence, scientists will have completed mapping the genetic code of human beings. The infamous Human Genome Project is no longer a science fiction dream proposed by Ray Bradbury or Arthur C. Clarke. It is also very likely that by the time you read this, a news headline will read that the first human has been cloned. Enter the brave new world!

For centuries, perhaps millennia, people have known that various physical traits as well as aspects of personality are passed down from generation to generation. This means that the good aspects as well as the less desirable factors may be shared. Human genetics is very complex. What we know is that some traits are pronounced (facial features), while others are recessive (such as eye color). The same is true for aspects of health. Current research suggests that various aspects of well-being are also passed through the genes. Keeping in mind that there are many factors involved with wellness, including hundreds of environmental aspects, not to mention psychological stress, let's take some time to look at your family tree.

Starting with your parents, then grandparents, and then moving on to offshoots such as your aunts, uncles, brothers, sisters, and finally great-grand-parents and anyone else you can reach out to, make a chart of your family and their health history. Start with the most obvious aspects (such as age) and note quality of health, any diseases (heart disease, diabetes, lupus, cancer, and so on), and cause of death if the person is no longer living. Although what you see when you start climbing your family tree won't explain your entire health history or your complete health status, it will begin to give you an idea of what direction you are headed.

If you are adopted, you may have to look a little harder to locate the roots of your tree. The dynamics of being adopted can be difficult at times, but not impossible.

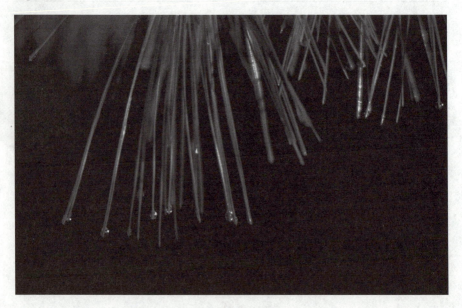

42. STRESS AND DISEASE

Stephanie is a wife of 13 years and a mother of three children. Her husband, Ted, is a sales representative for a large multinational corporation, which calls on him to travel four days of each week, sometimes more.

It's a tough job raising one kid, let alone three. It's a tougher job doing it alone. Despite her love for her husband, Stephanie will be the first to admit that she holds much resentment toward him and his job. This resentment has affected her health.

"Just look at me," she said one day. "I've lost three organs to stress—my appendix, gall bladder, and ovaries, and on top of that, I'm thirty pounds overweight. You better believe there has been a lot of stress in my life. Stress in the form of anger."

Researchers in the field of psychoneuroimmunology have long known of the stress and disease connection. Recent data suggest that as much as 80 percent of all disease and illness is stress related. Some would say this estimate is too conservative, that the percentage is actually much higher.

Today, the connection between stress and disease is more than an obvious one. We need to make ourselves aware of this connection so we can begin to resolve the issues that show up as colds, flus, back aches, migraines, ulcers, fever blisters, or hemorrhoids. Are you aware of any symptoms of disease or illness that you can trace to some unresolved emotions? Can you recall the event that precipitated the feelings? Please write about it here.

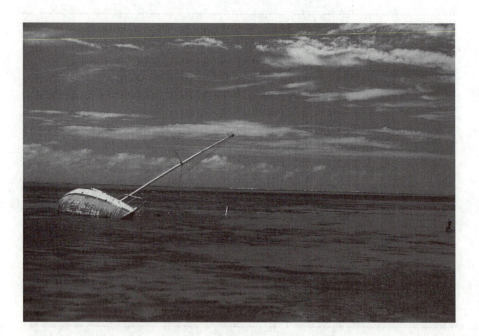

43. WHEN YOUR BIOGRAPHY BECOMES YOUR BIOLOGY

The cause of illness is ultimately connected to the
inner stresses present in a person's life.
Carolyn Myss

In the early 1980s Robert Ader coined the term *psychoneuroimmunology* to distinguish a new field of study, the field of mind–body medicine. What he and now countless others have discovered is that there is an amazing and profound connection between the mind and the body. To the contrary of French philosopher René Descartes, the mind and body are not separate entities. This means that our minds and the emotional thoughts we produce have an incredible impact on our physiology.

One person to emerge onto the stage of mind–body medicine is Carolyn Myss, Ph.D. A woman with an incredible ability to see what most others cannot, Myss has the gift to view a person's energy field and assist physicians in determining disease or the cause of a disease. Myss has a remarkable rate of accuracy, especially considering that she can do this from hundreds of miles away. First intrigued by the concepts of the human energy field and the chakras (spinning wheels of energy positioned over several major body organs from head to spine), Myss has focused her own energy into teaching people about the awareness of mind–body–spirit harmony.

In her most recent book, *The Creation of Health*, Myss discusses the idea that a life history, in terms of experiences, becomes intertwined with the cells of a body (Shealy and Myss, 1988). From hundreds of documented case studies, she has come to the understanding that symptoms of disease and illness don't start in the body; they end there. Can cervical cancer be rooted in sexual molestation? Can lower back pain be rooted in financial insecurities? Myss thinks so. Judging by her track record (95 percent accuracy), she stands on pretty solid ground.

According to Carolyn Myss, getting your life story out and examined is one of the first steps to optimal health. By means of coming to terms with your biography, you can release the negative energies that distort the integrity of each and every cell in your body. So what is your biography? What are some of the events that you now carry in the memoirs of each cell? Take some time to explore these and perhaps other life-long memories that may now be a part of your biology.

44. MY BODY'S RHYTHMS

The body has an internal clock that runs on a 24- to 25-hour day. If you were to lock yourself away from all the natural elements (sunlight, temperature fluctuations, etc.) and the grips of technology (e.g., TVs, radios, computers, etc.), as some people have for research purposes, your body would fall into a natural pattern, its *circadian rhythm.* To a large extent, these rhythms are based on and are strongly influenced by the elements of the natural world, the earth's rotation, the gravitational pull, the earth's axis, and several other influences we are probably not even aware of.

Other rhythms influence our bodies as well: *infradian rhythms* (less than 24-hour cycles) such as stomach contractions for hunger and rapid eye movement cycles, and *ultradian rhythms* (more than 24-hour cycles), such as menstrual periods and red blood cell formation.

It has been said that as we continue to embrace the achievements of high technology and separate ourselves even further from the reaches of nature, we throw off our bodies' natural rhythms. When these rhythms are thrown off for too long a time, various organs that depend on the regularity of these rhythms go into a state of dysfunction.

The college life holds no particular order for body rhythms. You can eat dinner one day at 6:00 P.M. and the next day at 9:30 P.M. We won't even talk about sleep! Perhaps at a young age your body can rebound from these cyclical irregularities. More likely than not though, regular disruptions in the body's rhythms will manifest quickly in various ways like irritability, fatigue, lack of hunger, restless sleep and insomnia, low resistance to illness, and lowered mental capacities.

1. What is your general sense of your body's rhythms?

2. Do you keep to a regular schedule with regard to eating, sleeping, exercise? Or does the time you do these vary from day to day?

3. How closely are you connected with nature? Do you spend time outdoors every day? Do you find yourself more tired, perhaps even more irritable as we shift from autumn into winter? Do you find yourself more energized, perhaps more positive or optimistic, as we shift from winter to spring?

4. If you are a woman, what is the regularity of your menstrual period? Can you identify a pattern with your nutritional habits, stress levels, and other daily rituals that may influence your menses?

45. HEALTH ORACLES

An oracle is a message from the future about various possibilities and probabilities. The future is never certain, but there are unique insights that may guide us toward our best interests. Oracles range from horoscopes and the Internet to tips on the stock market. This wisdom, or oracles, can come from a friend, a family member, a news headline, or some mystical experience, all of which serve the purpose of guiding you safely from point A to point B on the journey of human experiences.

In ancient Greece the most famous insights were sought from the Oracle of Delphi. Today, insights can come from just about anywhere. The key to oracles isn't so much where or from whom the insights come, but how adept we are at interpreting various messages that we take in through our conscious mind. To put it another way, keys to a car are great, but only if there is a car that the keys fit into.

So here is your assignment: In the next three days, be observant. Listen carefully to what people say regarding aspects of life that interest you, particularly your health. Expand your field of vision to include things that are often ignored or censored by your mind and, once again, observe. In the course of the next three days, come up with three oracles, three sources of information that are readily available to provide you information, insights, or intuitive thoughts to help solve any problems or issues you are currently dealing with.

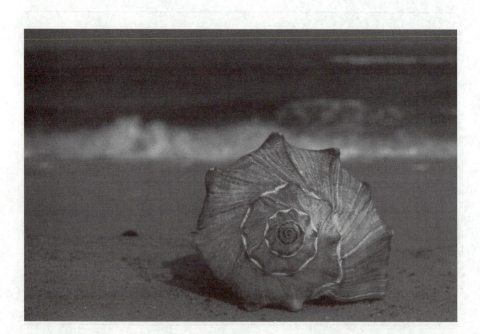

Oracles

1. _____

2. _____

3. _____

Insights

A. _____

B. _____

C. _____

Additional Comments

_____

_____

_____

_____

_____

46. ENERGY: THE LIFE FORCE

Look, and it cannot be seen. Listen, and it cannot be heard.
Form that includes all forms. Subtle beyond all conception.
Lao Tzu

There is a life force of subtle energy that surrounds and permeates us all. The Chinese call this force "chi." To harmonize with the universe, to move in unison with this energy, to move as free as running water is to be at peace with or to be one with the universe. This harmony of energy promotes tranquility and inner peace.

To understand the concept of chi, it is helpful to view it in the cultural perspective where it originated. Clinically speaking, the Chinese concept of health is quite different from that understood in the Western hemisphere. Unlike those in the West who view health as the absence of disease and illness produced by bacteria and viruses, the Chinese view health as an unrestricted current of subtle energy that runs throughout the body. When chi, the subtle energy that flows through the body in a network of meridians or "energy gates," is restricted or congested, the body is susceptible to physiological dysfunction. Hence, disturbances with the human energy field will result in physical symptoms of disease or illness.

According to Chinese medicine, it is not necessarily the bacterium or virus that causes physical dysfunction or disease; these are thought to be present everywhere. Rather, a state of poor health is thought to result from both internal and external factors, which ultimately do one in because of low resistance from non-harmonious (blocked) energy. Stated another way, these "pathogens" are constantly present; it is low resistance to them that makes one vulnerable to the disease. From a Chinese perspective, an unrestricted flow of energy helps maintain one's resistance to disturbing influences, be they biological, psychological, or sociological in nature.

Let's assume for a moment that the Chinese philosophy of health holds some merit, that a person's health status is based on the flow of energy. Perhaps you can gain a new perspective on your health from sensing your own energy levels. The following questions ask you to examine your energy level(s) as the underlying current of your health status.

1. What do you notice about your level of energy and your health status? For example, are there times when your energy is low, only to be followed by catching a cold or flu? Describe what you feel like when you are energized and compare it to when you feel drained of energy.

2. Do certain circumstances, events, or episodes seem to drain your energy? What are they? Do you see patterns here?

3. When you are feeling run down, as if you are running on empty, what do you do to recharge yourself?

4. In the Chinese culture, t'ai chi, acupuncture, and acupressure are used to equilibrate the body's energy levels, clear the meridians, and restore one to a sense of well-being. Have you tried one or more of these techniques? If so, what are your impressions? If not, would you consider giving one of them a try?

47. I HAVE A VISION: THE ART OF VISUALIZATION

A popular song back in the 1960s had a line that went like this: "Thinking is the best way to travel." In many ways this is true. The mind has an incredible ability to project itself to many places—some places the body might have been to, some only the mind visits in dreams.

Traveling on the thoughts generated by the mind, we can go anywhere. No ticket or baggage required, only a desire and imagination.

If you had the ability to project yourself anywhere, where you could relax for an hour or so, where would you go? This journal theme invites you to plan five mental minivacations, then use the powers of your imagination to take you there.

Visualization can also be used to heal the body by using your imagination to create a vision of restored health to a specific organ or region of your body. In fact, the role of visualization is one of the leading techniques in mind–body medicine.

The purpose of this journal theme is to sharpen your imagination and relaxation skills so that when you recognize you need to unwind you can escape, if only momentarily, to a place that gives you peace of mind. When drafting these images, give as much detail as possible so you can not only see them in your mind's eye, but actually feel yourself there through all five senses.

What are some healing visualizations you can use to restore yourself back to health?

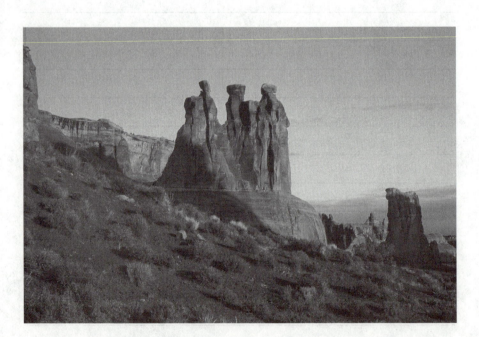

1.

2.

3.

4.

5.

V. UNHEALTHY CHOICES

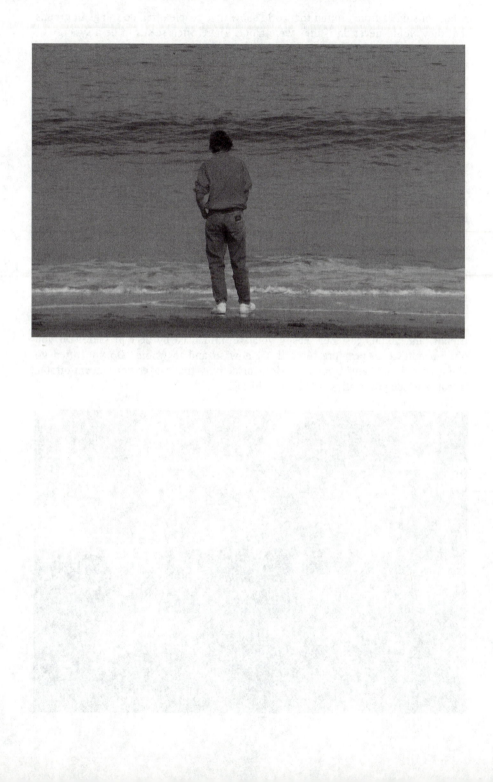

48. ME? PEER PRESSURE?

A host of studies from around the world show that people often do things in groups that they would never do if they were alone. There often seems to be a synergy of influence when a group of people collects. This synergy tends to pull everyone in, and to some extent, each person begins to conform to the group's desires. To stand up to, confront, or walk away from the group's influence may lead one to be mocked, ridiculed, or shunned. When self-esteem is vulnerable, ego boundaries are being stretched, and personality traits are becoming sharpened, to be shunned from your peer group is far harder to accept than the behavior of the group, even if it violates your morals.

In the early stages of the growth cycle, there is a craving to explore the world and experiment with our behaviors. And after all, this is a large part of the human journey. At some point in your life, you may puff on a cigarette, sip a shot of whiskey or scotch, or even take a hit on a joint to see what these experiences are like. The danger lies in getting caught up in the influences of others, even when we know the result is not in our best interest. There is a difference between taking a puff on a cigarette to see what it is like and lighting up to look cool.

Peer pressure has less to do with experimentation and discovery than with the issues of acceptance and rejection. It is human nature to want to be accepted by people we admire and respect. This desire to be accepted can lead us to actions and behaviors that compromise our integrity, morals, and our health.

This journal entry asks you to take a look at both your behaviors and your friends, and ponder just how easily you are influenced by peer pressure! Do you often acquiesce to peer pressure? If so, how so and to whom? Do you often go along with friends and agree to an idea or activity that makes you uncomfortable (because inside you really don't agree with it)?

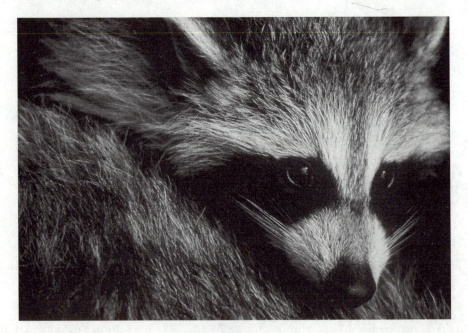

49. CHEERS!

It's hard to imagine that something that can taste so good initially can have such a bad aftertaste and potentially cause so many problems down the road. Be honest: most likely the first time you sipped a taste of beer, wine, or some other alcoholic beverage, you didn't think it tasted very good. But, as they say, alcohol is an acquired taste. Unfortunately what can also be acquired with alcohol is a series of problems that can ruin not only your own life, but also the life of practically everyone you come in contact with.

By the time you enroll in college, you have probably seen thousands of beer commercials, and have been subtly conditioned to the pleasures of drinking. It's well known that the problems with drinking usually start well before college, but it's during the college years where freedom to drink (legally or illegally) is when health habits become etched in stone. This is why so much attention is placed on peer education regarding the good, the bad, and the ugly of drinking in residence halls and all over campus.

Alcoholism isn't just a biochemical disease. The addiction to alcohol (and for that matter, all other substances) is holistic in nature, meaning that it's a disease of the mind, body, spirit, and emotions. And while there are certain people with a genetic disposition to alcoholism, treating this disease solely as a genetic disorder would be a disaster. Even if there are no known genetic causes, it is a well-known fact that people drink more when they are stressed—the connections among mind, body, spirit, and emotions run very deep.

The number of people with a drinking problem is grossly underestimated because of the shame associated with the disease. Most people deny they have a problem until well after the problem has consumed them. Current research indicates that each person with a drinking problem negatively affects ten people in their social circle: children, parents, friends, and work colleagues, not to mention those injured or killed in car accidents. In truth, we are all affected by the disease of alcoholism, either directly or indirectly.

Here are some thoughts to reflect upon regarding this topic:

1. Have you been affected by the wake of alcoholism, either through your parents, grandparents, aunts, uncles, siblings, or perhaps your own children? If so, how?

2. When did you have your first drink? When did you start drinking as a matter of habit? How much do you spend on alcohol per week?

3. Have you had a bad experience with alcohol (e.g., alcohol poisoning, car accident, drunk driver accident, date rape, physical abuse, sports riots, etc.)? If so, highlight the experience and describe your feelings about it.

4. Alcohol can be found in a great many products including cold remedies, herbal products, and mouthwashes. How aware are you of your alcoholic intake?

5. Alcohol is just one of many substance addictions. The process of denial, cover-up, and addictive behavior is the same with similar substances. Share your thoughts if you can relate to this.

6. Share any other comments you wish to write on this topic.

50. DO YOU SUFFER FROM AFFLUENZA?

God, all I ask is the chance to prove that money can't buy happiness.
Graffito at the University of Illinois

There is a disease going around the country that is known to be very infectious. To date there are no known antibiotics to cure it. The disease is called *affluenza*. No one really knows when it started, but it seems to have hit epidemic proportions in the mid-1990s and is still going strong. Fueled by a surging economy and an unbridled stock market, affluenza has become a disease to be reckoned with. No matter the state of economic affairs (good or bad), this disease is now ever-present.

Affluenza can best be described as an insatiable hunger for the good life, the rich life. Affluenza is the consumption of material possessions, hundreds and hundreds of material possessions. Some people call affluenza an addiction, because unlike a cold or flu, this disease doesn't go away in nine days. The purchase of clothes, CDs, DVDs, cars, and so on serves as a "fix" to lift one's self-esteem until the novelty has worn off and, poof, the process starts all over again. The problem is that buying these items to excess only strives to fill a void that can never be filled.

We live in a consumeristic society that rewards this behavior. Listen to people's conversations—within the first five minutes, someone will mention something they have bought.

Here are some questions to ponder and write about regarding the topic of affluenza:

1. What products have you bought in the past six months? Make a list.

2. Describe in detail how you feel after you make a big purchase in a store.

3. How often do you share the news of this purchase with your friends and family?

4. Do you see any relationships between the constant need to buy items and make purchases (retail therapy) and addictive behavior?

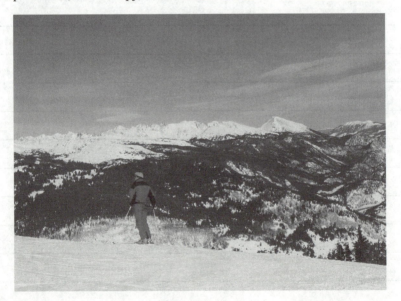

51. FREEDOM AND RESPONSIBILITY

It's a pity that the word *responsibility* wasn't in the phrase "life, liberty and the pursuit of happiness." Perhaps the idea of freedom with responsibility was so obvious, it only had to be implied. Perhaps it was inferred. We may never know, but what is often implied on one day is ignored or forgotten on the next. Such is the case with the concept of responsibility.

Freedom, or liberty, is a cornerstone of American culture. Responsibility should be, too. In truth, you cannot have one without the other. Each serves as a check and balance for the other. It was noted psychologist Viktor Frankl who once said that if we have a Statue of Liberty on the East Coast we should have a Statue of Responsibility on the West Coast to provide balance.

When we first leave home and head off to college, we assert independence with various freedoms to which we didn't have access under the rule of our parents. We may stay out later, we may sleep in longer, we may do a host of things we would never dream of doing at home. Freedom to do what we please is wonderful. But the flip side to freedom is responsibility; ultimately we are responsible for our every act, even if the consequences seem too distant or improbable to consider.

Such is the case with many reckless health behaviors (e.g. drinking, drugs, irresponsible sex). It seems sometimes that youth is a form of immortality, yet the illusion is a short-lived one. Every act of freedom carries responsibility. Freedom does not act in opposition to responsibility, but in collaboration with it.

Now ask yourself about your freedoms, your health behaviors, and your sense of responsibility about them. Please describe your feelings about these values and how they influence your choice of health-related behaviors.

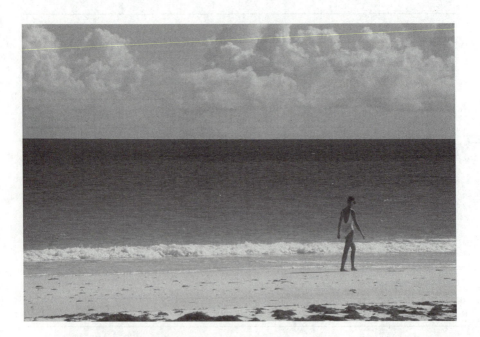

116

52. I HAVE NO SECRETS!

Secrets are the cornerstone of psychological dysfunction.
Gail S., recovering alcoholic

Everybody has a secret or two. There are things in our past that we really don't wish to share with the world. Typically, the things we keep secret are things that make us look bad. Relatives in prison, alcoholic parents, sexual abuse, and drug addictions are just a few of the more common skeletons in the closet, but there are hundreds more.

Here's the problem with secrets: They lead to emotional dysfunction. We try so hard to shove these bones to the back of the closet that they come back to haunt us. Addictions are the prime example of dysfunctional secrets.

Health experts agree that keeping secrets like this is anything but healthy. Having said that, you should know that there is a big difference between secrets and surprises. Secrets are typically things we are ashamed of and try to hide. Surprises are things we tend to hold back on until the appropriate time to acknowledge them. Examples of surprises include presents, engagements, pregnancies, and promotions.

The explanation of the difference between secrets and surprises may be a futile exercise in semantics, but the real message here is not to have any secrets within yourself. To do this, you must be really honest about yourself with yourself. So take some time to comb your mind and ask yourself whether you are keeping any secrets that are causing some level of dysfunction in your life. Are there some skeletons that need to be cremated?

Now is the time to do some cleaning of the closets. To keep a degree of security when you write about your secrets, feel free to use the third person so that you have the freedom to reveal the truth without feeling overexposed. Good luck!

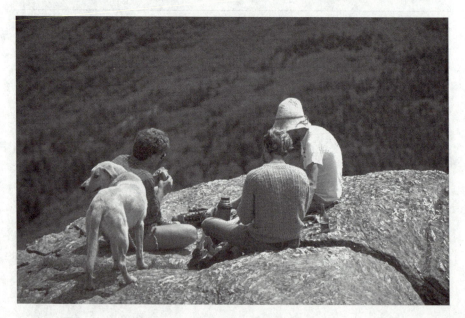

VI. MAKING HEALTHY CHOICES

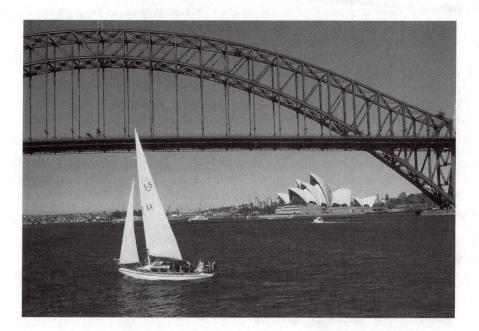

53. EXPLORING COMPLEMENTARY MEDICINE

In 1999 a revised study was published by the *New England Journal of Medicine* that stated that more than one-third of the American public partakes in the practice of complementary medicine. While this was no big surprise to the average citizen, it was disturbing news to the medical community, mostly because of the $20 billion a year spent on these types of therapies. Most, if not all, of that amount was out-of-pocket expense because insurance companies as a rule do not reimburse these types of healing modalities. Rather than be disturbed, medical professionals should have been delighted that such a large population of people had taken the initiative to be responsible for their own health care rather than having continued to take a passive role as has been the custom.

What we in this country call complementary is often referred to as traditional medicine in other parts of the world. Related forms of health care include, but are not limited to, acupuncture, herbal remedies, massage therapy, homeopathy, naturapathy, yoga, t'ai chi, music therapy, chiropractic medicine, flower essences, aromatherapy, art therapy, Rekei, and macrobiotic diets.

How do you feel about complementary medicine? Do you know anyone, family or friends, who have tried or use one or more forms of alternative therapies? Have you ever tried one or more of these types of therapies? If so, what was your experience? If not, would you consider trying some form for either a chronic health problem or as part of your health maintenance strategy? If you have not had any exposure, yet your curiosity is aroused, which of these listed or other complementary medical practices intrigues you?

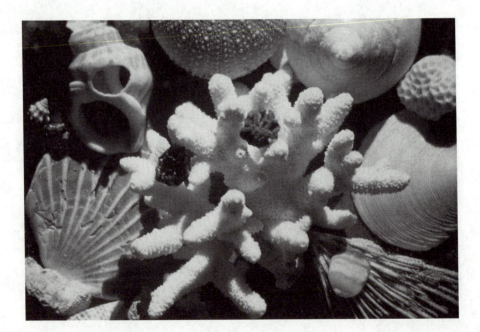

54. MY LOCUS OF CONTROL

The more you depend on forces outside yourself
the more you are dominated by them.
Harold Sherman

Several decades ago a psychologist named Julian Rotter presented the idea that there are two human drives—internal and external motivation. Rotter called them internal and external locus of control.

People who have an external locus of control tend to feel their lives are controlled by outside factors such as the weather, the stars, the government, destiny, and consequences beyond their own domain. Someone with an external locus of control places blame (or credit) on others for their misfortunes (or blessings). People in this category more likely than not see themselves as passive participants in life. An internal locus of control signifies a vantage point from which an individual sees the responsibility within himself or herself. He or she relies on inner strengths and resources. When faced with a problem or difficult situation, people with an internal locus of control stand up to adversity by themselves. They see themselves as having an active, not passive, role in their lives.

Most likely there are few people who epitomize either end of the spectrum, but we tend to gravitate toward one side or the other. In terms of health, a person with an external locus of control would blame a cold, headache, ulcer, or heart attack on somebody or something. Conversely, a person with an internal locus of control would assume responsibility for his or her health. As long as there is no undue guilt associated with it, this is something health-care professionals teach daily.

If you were to venture a guess, where would you see yourself on this continuum? Would you most likely see yourself with an internal locus of control or an external locus of control? Perhaps another way to word it is this: Are you easily motivated by trophies, medals, and horoscopes, or does your source of inspiration come primarily from within? Take a few minutes to ponder the concept of health-related locus of control and share your thoughts here.

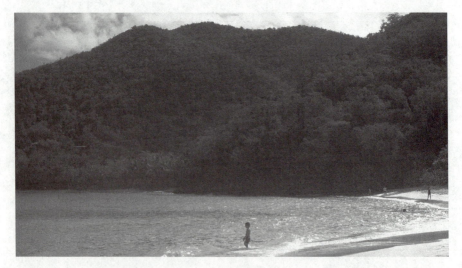

55. VOTING WITH YOUR WALLET

Are you a conscientious consumer? What this means is, how well do you know the companies that make the products you buy? The NIKE Corporation made national headlines a while back for allegedly paying substandard wages to their Asian workforce to ensure a bigger profit margin for their stockholders. Other multinational companies do the same thing. Although many companies give huge charitable donations to humanitarian efforts, they also reap enormous profits from their employees of third-world nations. Many Americans are oblivious to these facts until some media coverage makes it well known. Believe it or not, how you spend your money is a huge part of your overall wellness. Financial wellness means more than a balanced checking account. It means acting responsibly with your money. To act responsibly means being educated about where your money goes once it leaves your wallet, purse, or checkbook.

It is no exaggeration to say that we live in a fast and furious market economy. The buck rules! But we have a say in some of this. We buy the products from the companies that are often criticized for their workplace policies. These are the same multinational corporations that are said to have Congress and the president in their back pocket.

Ralph Nader has been an advocate for consumer protection for over forty years. Among many noteworthy efforts, he is credited with the mandatory installation of seat belts in all cars. Mr. Nader advocates a philosophy of voting with your checkbook. This is something you do anyway, but from now on, become more conscious of not only how you spend your money but also of who most benefits from the purchases you make.

Turn back to the very first journal theme regarding your personal health philosophy. Take a look at what you wrote and then spend some time to determine whether the money you spend supports or negates your health philosophy. If you are not sure of the companies you vote for with your checkbook, check them out on the Web.

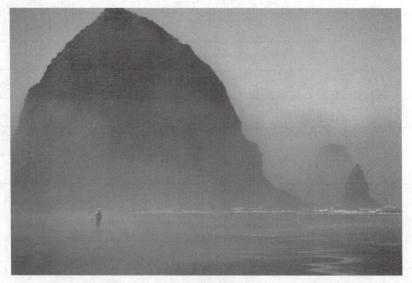

56. BEHAVIORS I'D LIKE TO CHANGE

If one desires change, one must be that change first
before that change can take place.
Gita Bellin

If you are like most people, you seek some type of self-improvement on a regular basis. Perhaps it's something you notice yourself doing. It may more likely be a suggestion from a friend, or worse, someone you aren't too particularly fond of. The most recognized time to make behavioral changes is January 1, when the year is new, the slate is clean, and the winds of change are in the air. Another time that we are reminded to make changes is on or around our birthdays, again a clean slate.

Two types of personalities and the respective behaviors linked with stress have now become household words: Type A and co-dependent. Type A behaviors include compulsive actions related to urgency, supercompetitiveness, and hostile aggression. These characteristics, primarily feelings of unresolved hostility, are thought to be closely associated with coronary heart disease. Co-dependent behaviors include perfectionism, overachievement, ardent approval seeking, control of others, inability to express anger and other feelings, ardent loyalty to loved ones, and overreactions. These types of behavior are now strongly linked to cancer.

Sometimes we are aware of our behaviors, but many times we are not. These actions are so ingrained in us that they are often second nature, so we seldom give them thought. Only when something we do is pointed out to us, or in an unguarded moment, do we see ourselves as perhaps others see us.

Behavioral psychologists have come to agree that changes are made first through awareness and then through motivation to change. But changing several habits at one time, which usually people try to do at the start of each new year, is very difficult, if not impossible. What is now commonly suggested is to try to change one behavior at a time. This way there is a greater chance of accomplishment. There is a progression of steps that, when followed, augment this process of behavioral change.

1. Become aware of your current behavior (e.g., biting my fingernails).

2. Find a new mindset to precede the new behavior you want to introduce (biting my nails is bad and I need to stop doing this).

3. Substitute a more desirable behavior in place of the old one (in the act of biting nails, stop and take a few deep breaths to relax).

4. Evaluate the outcome of trying the new behavior and renew or revise your plan and commitment (breathing helped, especially on that date last night; I'll keep trying this).

Sometimes it helps to write it down. Do you have any behaviors that you wish to modify or change? What are your options? Sketch them out here!

57. WHERE THERE'S A WILL, THERE'S A WAY!

One cannot discover new oceans until one has
the courage to lose sight of the shore.
Anonymous

Any great challenge that a person has overcome or dream that has been fulfilled required a combination of desire, determination, discipline, and willpower. Sometimes these are all included in the concept of willpower itself.

You may know several people who seem to have great willpower. They can eat one potato chip and stop. Or perhaps you know someone who has trained and successfully run a marathon. Willpower isn't a gift for a chosen few, it is a natural birthright for everyone. In a metaphorical sense, it is like a muscle. If we want to call on our willpower in times of challenge or to fulfill a dream, we need to exercise it on a regular basis.

1. On a scale of 1 to 10 (low to high), how would you rate your willpower? Subjectively, how do you feel about your level of willpower?

2. Do you have a challenge or goal that requires willpower to achieve a satisfying outcome?

3. What are some ways you could begin to strengthen your willpower muscle?

4. How can you use your willpower to shift from practicing an unhealthy behavior to a healthy one?

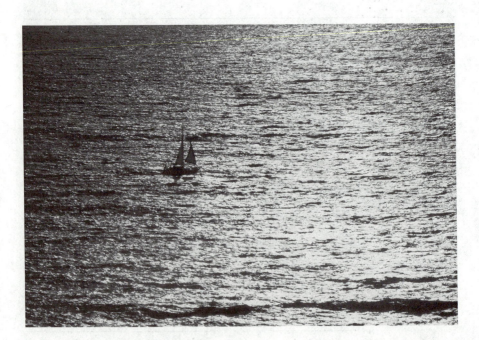

58. HEALTHY PLEASURES

In the book *Healthy Pleasures*, Robert Ornstein and David Sobel discuss the idea that in order to create a sense of balance in our lives, we need to remind ourselves to pat ourselves on the back, take responsibility for our moments of happiness, and engage in a host of behaviors that bring us a sense of joy and satisfaction.

Now you may say, "Hey, I already do this!" But most people don't, especially after they get out of college and get caught up in making money, paying bills, raising kids, and taking care of parents.

Healthy pleasures are just that, healthy. They don't cost much, either. To look at a sunset, to take an early morning walk in the woods, to treat yourself to an ice cream cone—these are healthy pleasures. How quickly they are forgotten when we feel stressed!

This journal entry asks you to list 25 healthy pleasures that you participate in on a regular basis. If you cannot come up with 25, list things you consider healthy pleasures that you intend to do soon.

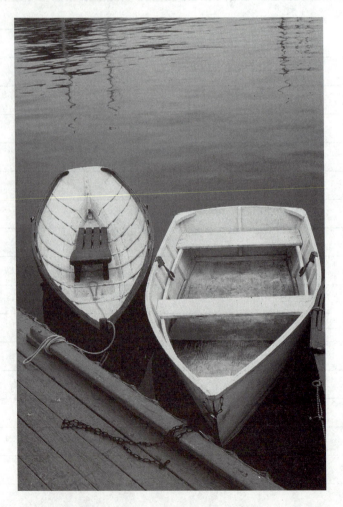

1.
2.
3.
4.
5.
6.
7.
8.
9.
10.
11.
12.
13.
14.
15.
16.
17.
18.
19.
20.
21.
22.
23.
24.
25.

VII. SPIRITUAL WELL-BEING

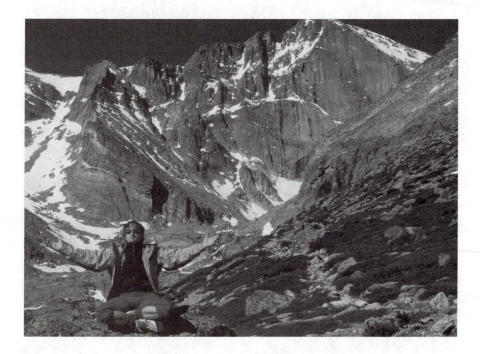

59. CONVERSATIONS WITH GOD

How come when we talk to God, its called praying,
but when God talks to us, it's called schizophrenia?
Lily Tomlin

Recently there has been much interest in the topic of spirituality, angels, miracles, and the healing power of prayer. It could be said that we in the American culture are going through a spiritual renaissance. One reason may be that after decades of materialistic pleasures, a large percentage of the baby-boom generation, as well as members of the so-called Generation X and "Millenium Generation," are coming up empty of any feeling of personal satisfaction. In essence, the value placed on material possessions has placed a wedge between a person and his or her divine self. So we find ourselves in a time of much spiritual hunger.

Although some people maintain that there is a distinction between the concepts of spirituality and religion, there is virtually no difference between those things spiritual and those things divine. Ideas of who or what God is may differ radically, but it is important only that you feel comfortable with your perceptions. Regardless of your conceptions, perceptions, beliefs, and attitudes, conversing with God, at some level, is the same as talking with your higher self. You might call this prayer.

Larry Dossey, M.D., has spent several years researching the concept of prayer. Like others before him who have taken a stab at understanding the divine nature of humanity, he has come to the realization that a prayer is merely a thought directed toward a power or energy that lies outside the domain of the five human senses, what Dossey calls the *non-local* mind.

Although several religions introduce one concept of prayer as a memorization of a poem (e.g., The Lord's Prayer, the Hail Mary) to be said in times of want or distress, this is just one of a host of ways to reach and speak to the God source that resides in and permeates all things. Prayer need not only be said in time of stress. This form of communication can be offered in times of joy and praise as well. Perhaps most important, prayer is an ongoing dialogue with your own thoughts, giving rise to the opportunity to elevate your level of consciousness, by realizing your connectedness to all things. So, in actuality, all thought has prayer potential.

Prayer also reflects your relationship with that part of you which is divine. This journal theme asks you to reflect on the spiritual aspect of your health and to continue this dialogue on paper.

60. MUSCLES OF THE SOUL*

Giving up is the final solution to a temporary problem.
Gerta Stein, Nazi concentration camp survivor

Just as a circle is a universal symbol of wholeness, so the butterfly is a symbol of the soul. Given the fact that butterflies, unlike the lowly caterpillar, have wings to fly, butterflies also are considered a symbol of transformation. They can rise above what was once a limiting existence. There is a story of a boy who, upon seeing a young butterfly trying to emerge from its chrysalis, tried to help by pulling apart the paper-like cocoon that housed the metamorphosis. The boy's mother, who saw what he was about to do, quickly stopped him by explaining that the butterfly strengthens its young wings by pushing through the walls of the cocoon. In doing so, its wings become strong enough to fly.

If you were to talk with anyone who has emerged gracefully from a difficult situation, they would most likely tell you that the muscles they used to break through their barrier(s) included patience, humor, forgiveness, optimism, humbleness, creativity, persistence, courage, willpower, and love. Some people call these qualities inner resources. I call them "muscles of the soul." These are the muscles we use to dismantle, circumnavigate, and transcend the roadblocks and obstacles in life. Like physical muscles, these muscles will never disappear; however, they will atrophy with disuse. We are given ample opportunity to exercise these muscles, yet not everyone does.

Using the butterfly illustration, write in the wings those attributes, inner resources, and muscles of the soul that you feel help you get through the tough times with grace and dignity, rather than feeling victimized. If there are traits you wish to include to augment the health of your human spirit, yet you feel aren't quite there, write them outside the wings and then draw an arrow into the wings, giving your soul a message that you wish to include (strengthen) these as well. Finally, if you have a box of crayons or pastels, color in your butterfly. Then hang it up on the fridge or bathroom mirror—someplace where you can see it regularly to remind yourself of your spiritual health and your innate ability to transcend life's problems, big and small.

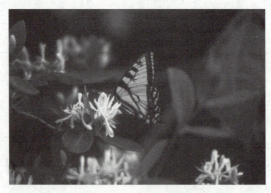

*"Muscles of the Soul" reprinted with permission, © 2000, Inspiration Unlimited.

HUMAN BUTTERFLY EXERCISE

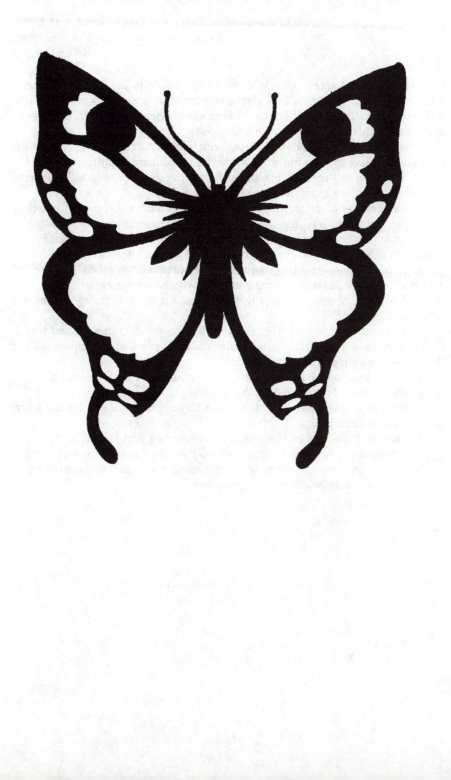

61. HEALTH OF THE HUMAN SPIRIT

We were born to make manifest the glory of God that is within us.
It's not just in some of us. It is in everyone.
Nelson Mandela

The health of the human spirit is wonderfully simple to achieve, yet at times equally difficult to maintain. It is simple because there are endless ways to make your spirit soar. It is difficult because it is so easy to get caught up in the day-to-day nonsense that keeps our spirits on the ground.

Aside from the process of centering, emptying, grounding, and connecting, there are several recipes for nurturing the health of the human spirit:

1. *The art of self-renewal:* Finding and practicing ways to re-energize yourself and taking time alone to restore your sense of who you are.

2. *The practice of sacred rituals:* Taking time to honor that part of ourselves and nature that comes from the divine essence of the universe.

3. *Embrace the shadow:* Acknowledging the dark side of our personality and learning to accept those parts of ourselves, even if we don't like them.

4. *Acts of forgiveness:* Learning to forgive ourselves and others who we feel have violated our humanness, learning to let go without resentment or shame.

5. *Surrender the ego:* Continually dismantling the walls of the ego to connect with your higher self.

6. *Compassion in action:* Remembering that we are all connected and love is the bond that ties us together. Acts of compassion have no other purpose than to share the expression of unconditional love.

7. *Living your joy:* Living in the moment with the idea that there are a host of experiences that can bring a smile to the face and joy to the heart.

8. *Keep the faith:* Knowing that there is a bigger game plan and you are a part of it. All things come in time.

9. *Hold an attitude of gratitude:* A habit of counting your blessings.

10. *Acceptance:* Accepting things that you have absolutely no control over.

Reflecting on these ten ideas, begin to address each one by commenting on how you engage in the health of your own spirit.

62. THAT'S THE SPIRIT!

We have all heard of school spirit, a sense of enthusiasm about the home team, whether it be football, basketball, or soccer. On a personal side, what do you do to pump up your self spirit?

We live in a culture where it is not typically advocated to pat yourself on the back and give yourself positive feedback. It is more likely that an internal voice constantly berates you, belittles you, and tells you that you're just not good enough. You're too fat, too thin, too skinny, too short, too tall, too whatever that seems critical to perfection.

In times like these (and there can be many), there needs to be a way to raise your spirits, boost your morale, and feel good about yourself. For sports teams we yell slogans, sing fight songs, and cheer at the top of our lungs. Why not do the same for ourselves? We can play on this theme and give ourselves affirmations.

1. Think of a phrase, slogan, word, or motto that you can say to yourself. Write it down, and learn to repeat it in times when you really need some wind in your sails.

2. List ten things that you can do to boost your morale and feel good about yourself.

3. List five people whom you consider to be role models, whom you admire for one or more traits. In your eyes, what makes them successful in life?

4. List five accomplishments that make you feel proud and remind you of your highest potential.

5. List ten of your positive attributes. If ten seems like too many, start with five.

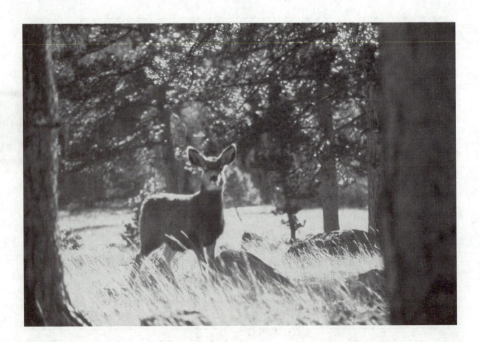

63. LIFE PASSAGES

How does a human pass through youth to maturity without breaking down?
Help from rites of passages at the most difficult stages.
Wendell Berry

Remember the first time you rode a bike by yourself without any help and how significant that was? Remember passing your driver's exam, or getting your first car? Remember your first real kiss, or the first time making love? Rest assured, life has many significant moments. But there are other kinds of moments. How about the day you found out your parents were getting divorced, the moment you learned of the death of a dear loved one, the day you lost your job, or the day you received the phone call that ended what was supposed to be the lifelong relationship with your soul mate?

These events on the human journey are often called life passages. In their own way, they are forms of initiation. We may not always remember the exact day that they happened, but good, bad, or ugly, we surely remember the experiences. Ageless wisdom suggests that if we can learn from these experiences then even the worst situations, in hindsight, are not so bad after all.

Some people get stuck in their life passages. They grow bitter and resentful about a situation and they carry that around for decades. In the age of Oprah, where we are all invited to do our "inner work," we now know that avoiding issues has a serious effect on all aspects of our health.

This journal theme asks only two questions:

1. What would you say is the most significant life passage you have experienced to date?

2. What did you learn from the experience?

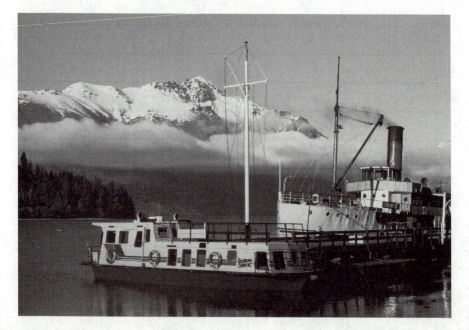

64. THE MEANING OF LIFE

*We had to teach disparaging men and we had to remind ourselves, that it did not
matter what we expected from life, rather what life expected from us.*
Viktor Frankl, Nazi concentration camp survivor

By far the most important question to ask ourselves is what is our purpose in life.
To seek and find the meaning of life is the cornerstone of spiritual wellness. So
often we journey through life looking to see what we can get out of our parents,
our education, our jobs, and our government. Perhaps we have it all wrong! It's not
what we can get out of life, it's what we give to life that makes life worth living.
This perspective inspired President John F. Kennedy to create the Peace Corps. It
also inspired him to say these now famous words: "Ask not what your country can
do for you. Ask what you can do for your country."

The college years are ripe to ask the question, What am I doing with my life?
This often happens when you ponder what major to select, or upon graduation you
realize this isn't the field you really want to be in. Asking yourself what your
purpose in life is, is searching to the depths of your soul. And it is a question that
must be asked with repeated frequency.

In your heart of hearts, what do you feel is your purpose in life? Why do you
feel this way? If you know what the answer is, and you can articulate why, the
next important question is, What is the best way to fulfill your life purpose so that
it is meaningful, and a significant contribution to humanity?

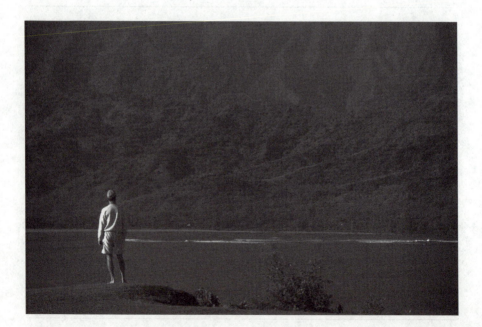

65. K-PAX REVISITED

In the spring of 2001, scientists documented the existence of at least 98 planets outside our solar system. Because of the Hubble Space Telescope, astronomers are having to readjust their perceptions of the universe to match the reality of space, now made more visible through advanced technology. It is interesting to note that when you were born, astronomers were discovering that what they thought were distant stars were actually remote galaxies. Since no one had ever seen a planet outside our solar system, it was conclusive that there must not be any! With newer space telescopes, now it's anyone's guess what we might find out there. This may sound like a cliché, but what was science fiction yesterday is quickly becoming reality today.

It is very likely that within your lifetime, and it could be as soon as the next few years, the CNN news headlines will reveal that humans have encountered intelligent life outside the planet. Given the fact that we know that there are several planets out there, and most likely several million more, the existence of life is more probable now than ever before.

Futurists at companies such as Ball Aerospace suggest, based on the current findings, that our discovery of extraterrestrial life is just around the corner. There is no doubt that while many people eagerly await the news that we are not alone in the universe, there are some people who will be pretty shaken by this. Others will simply deny it. In the movie *K-Pax*, the audience was left with the decision of whether the protagonist was an alien or simply delusional.

What exactly do extraterrestrials have to do with health? The possibilities are endless! But rather than diving back into science fiction, it would be a good idea to establish your thoughts on this right now. Are you the kind of person who already knows we are not alone in the universe, or are you very sure that we are the closest thing to intelligent life for galaxies around? What impact do you think a discovery such as this would have on the world population as a whole? What about Americans? What about you and your family? You don't have to be a fan of *The X-Files* or *Star Trek* to write about your thoughts and feelings of life outside the planet Earth. Merely living on earth right now makes you qualified.

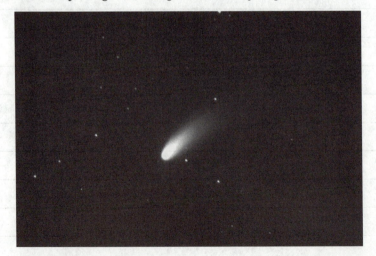

66. MY INNER RESOURCES

Be humble for you are made of earth.
Be noble for you are made of stars.
Serbian Proverb

If our collection of life experiences can be compared to that of a journey, then the problems, issues, difficulties, and dilemmas we encounter on that journey (which at times seem to halt our progress) can likewise be compared to roadblocks on the human path.

When a roadblock befalls the traveler on a trail in the wilderness, the course of action he or she takes depends on the tools and resources at hand. Obstacles can be climbed over, ducked under, skirted around, sawed through, blown up, and with an about-face, perhaps avoided.

Obstacles we encounter are neither fallen trees nor boulders. Nor can the roadblocks we face on life's journey be sawed through or blown up. In reality, the challenges faced on life's sojourn come to us in the likes of alcoholic parents, financial debt, rebellious children, or the death of a spouse or close friend. In essence, they must be resolved and transcended. It is the only way.

Remember the story of Dorothy and the Wizard of Oz? This is a classic story of obstacles and inner resources. Dorothy's desired destination was to return home; the roadblock on her journey was the witch. The scarecrow, tin man, and lion were personifications of her inner resources—intellect, compassion, and courage, respectively.

Consider for a moment the concept of inner resources. Comprised of traits that help us get through the tough times in our lives, they assist us to resolve and transcend whatever has been put in front of us, to lend integrity to our human spirits. Humor, creativity, passion, willpower, courage, patience, and faith are examples of special qualities that we can and often do use in troubled times. Let's take a look at your inner resources.

1. What obstacles are you facing right now in this leg of your human journey? Rather than just list them, take some time to flesh out the details of each one.

2. We all have inner resources, but not all of us make use of the same ones. Whether you call these talents, gifts, or special abilities, list the inner resources that help you dismantle and resolve the roadblocks you listed above. Are there any you feel are missing that would help you on your journey?

3. Inner resources can be compared to muscles, and like muscles, atrophy with disuse or increase in size with some resistance. Now is the time to ask yourself which of your inner resources you have allowed to atrophy to a point where they are no longer functional. Next ask yourself, "What can I do to regain and strengthen these inner resources?"

67. THINGS I TAKE FOR GRANTED

Love wholeheartedly, be surprised, give thanks and
praise—then you will discover the fullness of life.
David Steindl-Rast

Almost instinctively, humankind has given thanks since they first set foot on earth. From animal sacrifices to banquet feasts to silent moments of praise, showing appreciation for the smallest of gifts or life's greatest pleasures is very much a part of the human condition. A unique tradition was established on the shores of the New World several hundred years ago when English immigrants and Native Americans sat down to perhaps the most famous autumn feast ever created, Thanksgiving. Appropriately, thereafter it became a yearly event.

It is easy to give thanks and praise in times of joy and happiness. It is rarely thought of, however, in times of crisis. Stress can produce some very ungrateful attitudes. Stressful events tend to cloud the mind with thoughts of frustration and anguish, some directed inward, most directed outward, and these can leave little room for much else. When the Pilgrims sat down to the first turkey dinner, times were hard. They had no indoor plumbing, no drug stores, no credit cards, and no daycare centers. Life was a real challenge. But in that challenge, life was reduced to the simplest of terms. The challenge was survival. In our day and age, survival is pretty much a given fact. The question isn't "Will I survive?" but rather "How well can I live?" Although theoretically the high-tech age has improved the quality of life, it also seems to drag with it pressures that negate this standard of quality.

More stress and less time to enjoy life's simple pleasures can make it difficult to give adequate time to sit back every now and then and appreciate the little things that make life special. Stress can blind vision. By consciously taking the blinders off, we can see the whole picture in better focus. Taking things for granted is as much a part of human nature as giving thanks. But so often, "we don't know what we've got 'til it's gone." A list of things that you take for granted could be endless, but start with 10 things. If you were to stop and think for a moment about some of them, just what would they be and why?

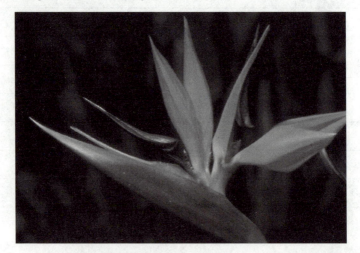

1. _____

2. _____

3. _____

4. _____

5. _____

6. _____

7. _____

8. _____

9. _____

10. _____

Additional Thoughts
_____

_____

_____

_____

_____

_____

_____

_____

_____

_____

_____

_____

_____

68. THE SECRET OF LIFE

I once took a ride with a pilot on a two-person harness paraglider. It was amazing, not to mention breathtaking! Gliding in the air for nearly an hour, my pilot told me that after looking for what seemed like an eternity, he found the secret of life. I asked him what it was, but he said he couldn't tell me—it was a secret. Then he laughed. As it turns out, he did tell me. And the secret of life is no secret at all. Why is something that inspires the very core of our existence hidden from view at nearly every turn? Perhaps it is that we are constantly bombarded with so many distractions that we walk around as if we had some kind of amnesia. Even before I took that ride that day, I discovered the secret of life myself. I could tell you what it is, but then it wouldn't be a secret!

The secret of life isn't something to learn from someone else, it's something to discover all by yourself. It may take days; it may take decades. Everyone is different. The secret to life has to do with an inner source of happiness and contentment, but it doesn't stop there. So what do you think the secret of life is? And once you find out what it is, how do you achieve it?

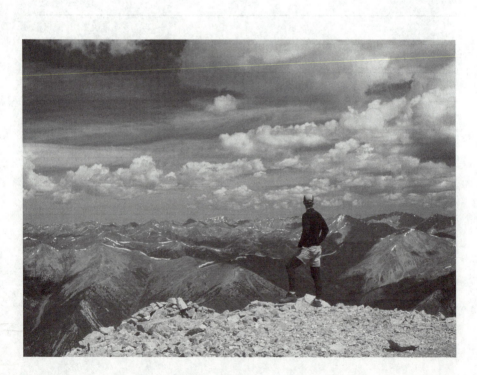

VIII. OVERCOMING OBSTACLES

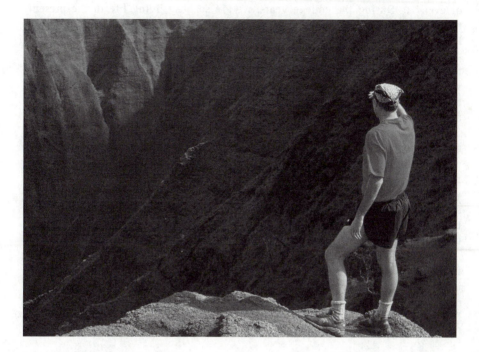

69. WHEN I'M 64

At the age of 20 or 30, it is hard to think what our lives will be like at age 50, 60, or even 70. During the college years, we are so busy living life in the present moment that to project ourselves 40 years ahead is not a common thought. In the late teens and early twenties, we actually feel immortal, as if we can live forever, and many of our behaviors reflect this. In fact, many of our behaviors are based on the idea that we can risk dealing with any problem later down the road, but today we will live for the moment. Although living in the present moment of our thoughts is greatly encouraged in some regards, living in the moment can also result in some pretty reckless behaviors.

Use your imagination for a few moments. Through the gift of imagination, you can wonder, "What if I were now 60 years old?" If you visit your grandparents or do some community work where you come in contact with senior citizens, you might pause and wonder what it must be like to be that old. As the thought goes, if we can project our thoughts ahead, we can chart the course of our lives by heeding some of the cautions. If you were to sit and talk with several senior citizens, the topic of health would surface quickly, probably within five minutes. If only I had done things differently when I was your age, the voices of wisdom tell us.

Imagine. What do you think you will be like at the age of 70? How will your health be? Will you still be able to do the things then as you do now if your health behaviors remain the same?

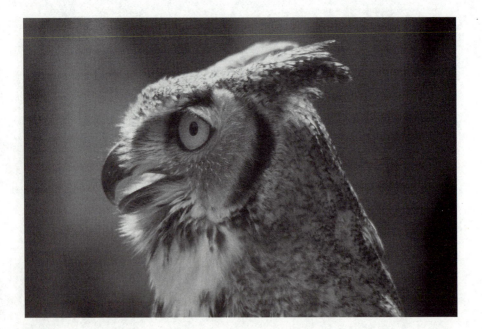

70. YOUR LAST WILL AND TESTAMENT

You can't take it with you, and where you are going,
you probably won't need it anyway.
Anonymous

This might be a good time to settle accounts. Over 60 percent of the American public does not have a will. Some people find the topic rather morbid, while it is fair to say that others are in a state of denial about their mortality. It would be really nice if all your worldly possessions would simply go automatically to those loved ones left behind; however, without proper action, the government steps in and takes their share first, leaving months, if not years, of legal hassles behind to sort everything out.

Although these next few pages won't serve as an official will, they will serve as a starting point to get the ball rolling. Start by making a list of your possessions (e.g., car, computer, DVD player, CDs, and books). Add to this any other items of value such as savings accounts, stocks, bonds, and mutual funds, if you have them. Just as your list of possessions will change through the years, so too will those to whom you wish to leave these items. But if you don't assign each item to a loved one, it's as good as gone. So indicate who gets what even if you decide to change your mind next year. Don't forget pets. If you have any children under the age of 18, specify who you wish to have look after them. Some people actually write notes or letters to their loved ones (a last goodbye of sorts) and have these passed out at the reading of the will. Finally, give some thought as to whether you would like to be buried or cremated, and where is it you wish your remains to go. Don't forget organ donation!

You might also wish to include a sentence or two about a living will and who you would like to assign "power of attorney" to in the event you couldn't make sound decisions for yourself.

Use the following page to start the process. At some point (sooner rather than later) transfer this to some letterhead stationery, make a few copies (for parents, kids, etc.), and have these notarized.

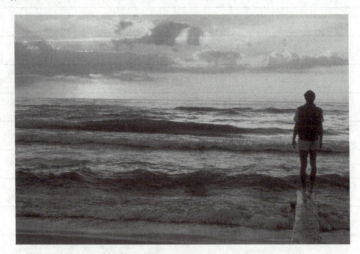

My Last Will and Testament

71. FORTY-EIGHT HOURS LEFT TO LIVE

Seek not hours to kill, but hours to live.
Kahlil Gibran, *The Prophet*

Many of us will never know the exact time of our death. Unlike the estimated time of our arrival here on earth, our departure is a little less exact.

There is an expression that states: Live each day as if it were your last! This means to live life with no regrets—to attend to all one's thoughts, wishes, and desires so as to make the human experience as rich as possible. Most certainly, there are some precautions to observe regarding this proverb. If we live each day on the edge, then most likely we will have a short life span. Rather than taking uncalculated risks, living each day as if it were your last is an invitation to live life to the fullest.

Author and lecturer Steven Levine asks this question: "If you had 24 hours to live, how would you spend your last day on earth?" After he has asked people this question and given them sufficient time to answer, he then asks, "What are you waiting for?"

Let's assume that you need more than 24 hours. Let's double it and make it 48 hours. How would you spend your last two days on the planet Earth? What would you see, who would you visit, what would you eat, who would you call? What would you do to make peace in your heart and leave with a smile on your face? Write about it here.

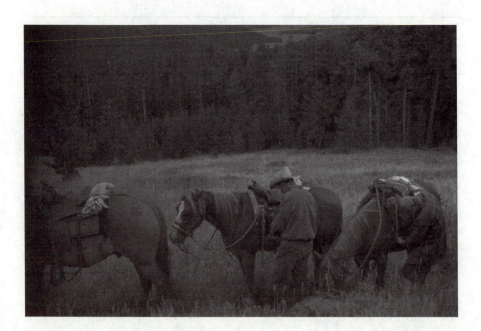

72. TERRORISM IN THE TWENTY-FIRST CENTURY

Let's roll!
Last recorded words of passenger Todd M. Beamer
on September 11, 2001, during his efforts to retake
Flight 93 from the terrorists over
Shanksville, Pennsylvania.

September 11, 2001, will be a date that lives in the minds of Americans forever. The devastating sight of the World Trade Center towers collapsing in seconds is embedded in our psyches and souls forever.

Ask anyone in Oklahoma City or students attending Columbine High School and they will tell you that September 11 wasn't the first episode of terrorism on U.S. soil. Yet the events on that day, with thousands of deaths, were unparalleled in the history of America. Once protected by the waters of the Atlantic and Pacific Oceans, the United States has now become as vulnerable as the rest of the world, experts say. Terrorism must now be considered a fact of life for most Americans on our own home soil.

A woman who survived the ordeal in New York City said that panic is not an option for dealing with terrorism. "The second you give into fear, you have given over your power and the terrorists have won." The fear of terrorism can lead to paranoia, which is about as unhealthy as the Ebola virus.

Here are some thoughts to ponder and reflect as well as some questions to answer on this topic:

1. What were your feelings the moment you learned of the events of September 11 (or any other similar day of terrorism)?

2. What thought(s) went through your mind as you saw the collapse of the World Trade Center towers?

3. There are many types of terrorism. Have you ever been subjected to terrorism, either at home or abroad?

4. Any additional comments you wish to share here?

73. HONORING MOTHER EARTH

Let us think of Mother Earth.
Native American Prayer

It is no overstatement to say that the planet Earth is in trouble! It is sick and desperately fighting for survival. Water and air pollution, nuclear waste dumps, holes in the ozone, deforestation, and the incredible rate of extinction of plants and animals—the telltale signs are everywhere. All you need to do is listen to the news or read a magazine and these stories jump out and smack you across the face.

It may seem hard to believe that the earth is a living entity. Western thought, so heavily grounded in the scientific ideology, makes this idea seem pagan at best. But if you were to listen to the Wisdom Keepers of the earth's indigenous peoples, you would hear that the notion of the earth as a living entity is sacred, not foolish or ludicrous. It is a simple truth. Even the ancient Greeks believed this, naming Mother Earth *Gaia*. Humans, once so close to the energies of the earth, have now grown very distant and separate from them. From air-conditioned bedrooms to the automobile, we have become slaves to the benefits of technology. It is not uncommon to hear people say that technology can fix what technology has damaged, which in essence puts human capabilities above the powers of the earth and sky. In the profound words of Chief Seattle, "All things connect. Man did not weave the web of life, he is merely a strand in it. Whatever he does to the web, he does to himself."

Sometimes in the cyclone of daily hassles and catastrophic events of our lives, we become disconnected from the natural elements that surround us. Whether or not we realize it, like a web, we are strongly connected to the earth. Despite all the wonderful advances in technology, we are still very dependent on the fruits and sustenance that Mother Earth provides and the cycles in which she turns. *Stress* has recently been defined as being separated or disconnected—disconnected from our friends, family, and the earth that sustains us. Inner peace is synonymous with connection and harmony with all. Therefore, part of the strategy to reduce stress is to reconnect with the planet we call home. Perhaps it's true that we can't change the world, but we can change a part of it by our interaction with it. This idea is summed up quite nicely in the slogan "Think globally, act locally."

Do some soul-searching with your Mother Earth in mind. If this concept is something you have never given serious thought to, now is the time to get serious, and not in a stressful way either. Here are some questions you can ask yourself to get the ball rolling:

1. How would you best describe your relationship with the planet Earth?

2. Do you see the earth as a rock spinning in space, or as a living entity that provides sustenance in one form or another to all her species of flora and fauna?

3. Getting back to nature can take many forms, from gardening to exotic vacations. What do you do to get back to nature when the urge strikes?

4. Biological rhythms and circadian variations are constant reminders that the earth strongly influences us. Are you in touch with these rhythms and, if not, why?

5. Any good relationship takes work. If so inclined, what steps do you feel you can take to enhance your relationship with Mother Earth?

74. ENVIRONMENTAL HAZARDS

We are a part of the natural world, even though it seems that many people never leave the confines of their home, car, or office in the course of a normal day. When factors such as population density, synthetic building materials, and electromagnetic waves are combined, the results can greatly affect the state of our health and well-being.

Environmental hazards go well beyond air and water pollution, although those are problems enough. Environmental hazards also go well beyond the detection of radon in your basement. Toxic materials used in the construction of homes, as well as the petrochemicals used in things such as cosmetics, deodorant, hair gel, and the like, are now thought to be directly related to, if not specifically responsible for, many chronic illnesses.

Take a look around your environment and carefully study the makeup of your surroundings. Make a list of those things that directly affect your life that you have suspicions about. For example, did you know that 69 percent of pregnant women who use an electric blanket suffer from miscarriages? The new worry is the alarming rate of brain tumors and cell phone use. (For a good resource on electromagnetic pollution, read *Cross Currents* by Robert Becker, published by Tarcher Books.)

Then consider how much time you spend in the natural world, the outdoors. How many minutes of sunlight do you get—enough to make vitamin D with your skin? Do some research and determine the quality of your drinking water. Current research suggests that our water contains increasing traces of antibiotics that people throw away down the drain.

This journal entry is designed to get you to think about your relationship to your environment and the steps you can take to improve this relationship. So, try to come up with twelve ways to cultivate this relationship.

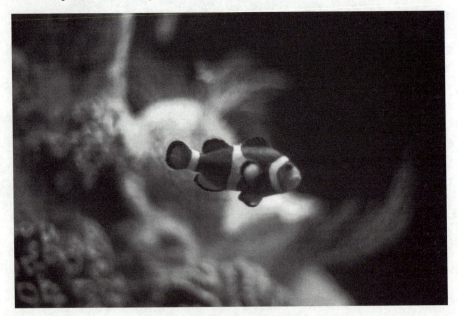

1. _____

_____

2. _____

_____

3. _____

_____

4. _____

_____

5. _____

_____

6. _____

_____

7. _____

_____

8. _____

_____

9. _____

_____

10. _____

_____

11. _____

_____

12. _____

_____

75. COPING WITH CHANGE

The only person who likes change is a wet baby.
Roy Blitzer

Most people don't like change. Oh sure, we like new music, new foods, and new clothes, but we hate it when our favorite radio station changes formats. We get pissed when our favorite TV show gets cancelled. And we are not too crazy about car accidents, divorces, being laid off from work, or having someone close to us die.

The reason we don't like change is that change tends to disrupt our comfort zones. Change comes in and moves things around, so much so that we get flustered, perhaps even angry. Most people would rather face the demons they know than the ones they don't know. Change begins with fear of the unknown, and it quickly develops into frustration and anger.

There are scores of bad ways to deal with change. They include some of our biggest health issues today: drinking, drug abuse, spousal abuse, and, of course, depression. Each of these ways doesn't really deal with the issues and concerns. If anything, these measures are acts of avoidance and only perpetuate the problem.

There are good ways to deal with change. People do it all the time. Lance Armstrong (cancer), Rosa Parks (civil rights), and the scores of people who lost loved ones in New York, Washington, D.C., and Pennsylvania on September 11 all come to mind.

Now is the time to use some foresight and harness your resources when the winds of change start blowing in your direction. Compose a list of ten effective ways to cope with change—any change that awaits you on the human journey. Here is an example to get you started:

Information seeking: Look for ways to get as much information about the events as possible so that the unknown becomes the known.

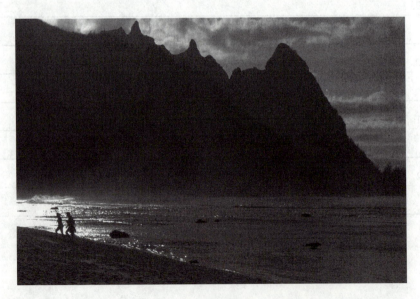

170

1. _____

_____

2. _____

_____

3. _____

_____

4. _____

_____

5. _____

_____

6. _____

_____

7. _____

_____

8. _____

_____

9. _____

_____

10. _____

_____

IX. REFLECTIONS

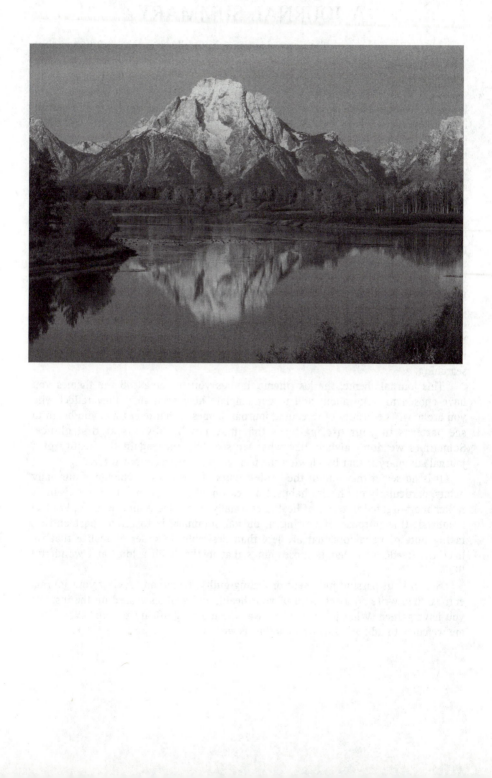

76. REFLECTIONS:
A JOURNAL SUMMARY

The underlying premise of wellness is that each person must
take responsibility for his or her own health.
Jon Robison, Ph.D.

When you take a look in the mirror, you see a reflection of yourself. You see an image (actually a reverse image) of your physical self. From an early age we get in the habit of checking our looks in the mirror. We check our hair, our skin, our teeth, our eyes, our clothes, our muscles—the works! A mirror image never tells us where we are going, only where we have been. The reflection that looks back is a composite of all that we are and all that we have become. A reflection is a snapshot of ourselves, much like a photograph.

The image in the mirror only represents the physical aspects. It tells very little, if anything, about our mental, emotional, and spiritual health. Sometimes a mirrored reflection doesn't even hint at physical problems. But there are other ways to determine these reflections. The journey you have taken through this journal workbook represents an image too—an image of your thoughts, feelings, attitudes, perceptions, opinions, and philosophies. Just as much as our physical attributes, and perhaps even more, these shape who we are as human beings.

This collection of journal themes represents an image of your health and well-being. The clarity of the image is only as good as that which you have chosen to reveal about yourself, which is why honesty is paramount when it comes to soul-searching.

This journal theme, the last theme, invites you to reread all the themes you have chosen to write about and to contemplate how accurately they reflect who you are now. The beauty of rereading journal themes is that over time, you begin to see patterns in your life, patterns that may not be obvious at first glance. Sometimes we don't always like what we see, but once again the beauty of a journal summary is that by viewing the past you can redirect your future.

It is no secret that one of the hardest parts of our lives to change is our daily habits, particularly our health habits. One reason why this is so is that our vision is rather short-sighted in terms of health, especially in our teens and twenties. We feel immortal! One purpose of writing a journal summary is to reread past entries, taking note of behaviors that are less than desirable, in order to realize that we have the freedom to change those things that might derail a long and wonderful life.

So, without passing judgment or feeling guilty, reread and review your journal entries, then write an assessment of your health and wellness based on the insights you have gained. What journal theme was the most significant to you? Why? You are welcome to add any further thoughts as well.

JOURNAL-WRITING RESOURCES

Abbott, H.P., *Diary Fiction: Writing as Action.* Cornell University Press, New York, 1984.

Abercrombie, B., *Keeping a Journal.* Margaret K. McKelderry Books, New York, 1987.

Adams, K., *Journal to the Self.* Warner Books, New York, 1990.

Baldwin, C., *One to One: Self-Understanding Through Journal Writing.* M. Evans, New York, 1977.

Britton, J., Burgess, T., Martin, N., McLeod, A., and Rosen, H., *The Development of Writing Abilities.* Macmillan, London, 1975.

Buzan, T., *Use Both Sides of Your Brain.* E.P. Dutton, New York, 1983.

Capacchione, L., *The Creative Journal: The Art of Finding Yourself.* Swallow Press, Athens, GA, 1979.

DeVota, Bernard (Ed.), *The Journals of Lewis and Clark.* Houghton Mifflin, Boston, 1953.

Dinesen, I., *Out of Africa.* Random House, New York, 1983.

Foster, S., with Little, M., *The Book of the Vision Quest: Personal Transformations in the Wilderness.* Prentice-Hall, New York, 1988.

Fulwiler, T (Ed.), *Journals Across the Disciplines.* Northeast Regional Exchange, Chelmsford, MA, 1985.

Goldberg, N., *Writing Down the Bones.* Shambhala Publications, Boston, 1986.

Hagan, K.L., *Internal Affairs: A Journal Keeping Workbook for Self-Intimacy.* Escapadia Press, Atlanta, GA, 1988.

Holly, M.L., *Writing to Grow: Keeping a Personal/Professional Journal.* Heinemann Educational Books, Portsmouth, NH, 1989.

Kaiser, R.B., The way of the journal. *Psychology Today,* 15:64–65, 1981.

Leedy, J.L., *Poetry Therapy: The Use of Poetry in the Treatment of Emotional Disorders.* J.B. Lippincott, Philadelphia, 1969.

Mallon, T., *A Book of One's Own: People and Their Diaries.* Ticknor and Fields, New York, 1984.

Mayer, H., Lester, N., and Pradl, G., *Learning to Write, Writing to Learn.* Boynton/Cook, Portsmouth, NH, 1983.

Morrison, M.R., *Poetry as Therapy.* Human Sciences Press, New York, 1987.

Pennebaker, J.W., *Opening Up: The Healing Power of Confiding in Others.* William Morrow, New York, 1990.

Progoff, I., *At a Journal Workshop.* Dialogue House Library, New York, 1975.

——, *The Practice of Process Meditation.* Dialogue House Library, New York, 1980.

Rainer, T, *The New Diary.* J.P. Tarcher, Los Angeles, 1978.

Rico, G.L., *Writing the Natural Way.* J.P. Tarcher, Los Angeles, 1983.

Seaward, B.L., *Managing Stress: Principles and Strategies for Health and Well-Being* (3rd ed.). Jones and Bartlett, Boston, 2002.

Simons, G.F., *Keeping Your Personal Journal.* Ballantine/Epiphany, New York, 1978.

Woodward, P., Howard, P., *Journal Jumpstarts: Quick Topics and Tips for Journal Writing.* Cottonwood Press, 1991.

REFERENCES

Allgeier, E., and Allgeier, A., *Sexual Interactions* (4th ed.). D.C. Heath, Lexington, MA, 1995.

Andreas, S., and Falkner, C. (Eds.), *NLP: The New Technology of Achievement*. Quill Books, New York, 1994.

Ayres, A. (Ed.), *The Wit and Wisdom of Mark Twain*. Harper & Row, New York, 1987.

Baum, E., *The Wizard of Oz*. Random House, New York, 1986.

Beattie, M., *Codependent No More*. Harper/Hazelden, New York, 1987.

——, *Beyond Codependency*. Harper/Hazelden, New York, 1989.

Becker, R., *Cross Currents*. Tarcher Press, New York, 1990.

Black Elk, W., and Lyons, W., *Black Elk*. Harper, San Francisco, 1990.

Borysenko, J., *Minding the Body, Mending the Mind*. Bantam Books, New York, 1984.

Boyd, D., *Rolling Thunder*. Delta, New York, 1974.

Branden, N., *The Six Pillars of Self-Esteem*. Bantam Books, New York, 1994.

Buscaglia, L., *Love*. Fawcett Crest, New York, 1972.

——, *Living, Loving & Learning*. Fawcett Books, New York, 1982.

Casey, K., and Vanceburg, M., *The Promise of a New Day*. HarperCollins, New York, 1983.

Catacchione, L., *The Creative Journal, The Art of Finding Yourself*. Swallow Press, Athens, GA, 1979.

De Graaf, J., Wann, D., Naylor, T., *Affluenza: The All-Consuming Epidemic*. Berrett-Koehler Publishers, San Francisco, 2001.

Dossey, L., *Healing Words: The Power of Prayer and the Practice of Medicine*. HarperCollins, New York, 1993.

Dyer, W., *Your Erroneous Zones*. Avon Books, New York, 1976.

Fanning, P., *Visualization for Change*. New Harbinger, Oakland, CA, 1988.

Foster, S., with Little, M., *The Book of the Vision Quest*. Prentice-Hall, New York, 1988.

Frankl, V., *Man's Search for Meaning*. Pocket Books, New York, 1984.

Gibran, K., *The Prophet*. Alfred A. Knopf, New York, 1981.

Hall, C., *A Primer of Freudian Psychology*. Mentor Books, New York, 1954.

Hayward, S., *A Guide for the Advanced Soul*. In-Tune Books, Avalon, Australia, 1984.

Jampolski, G., *Love Is Letting Go of Fear*. Celestial Arts, Berkeley CA, 1979.

Jung, C.G., *Man and His Symbols*. Anchor Press, New York, 1964.

——, *Mandalas of Symbolism*. Princeton University, Princeton, NJ, 1973.

Klein, A., *The Healing Power of Humor*. J.P. Tarcher, Los Angeles, 1989.

Kübler-Ross, E., *Death, The Final Stage of Growth*. Touchstone, New York, 1987.

Lerner, H., *The Dance of Anger*. Harper and Row, New York, 1985.

Lindbergh, A.M., *Gift from the Sea*. Vintage Books, New York, 1978.

Maltz, M., *Psycho-Cybernetics*. Pocketbooks, New York, 1960.

Martz, H., *If I Had to Live My Life Over Again, I Would Pick More Daisies*. Paper Mâché Press, Watsonville, CA, 1993.

Maslow, A., *The Farther Reaches of Human Nature*. Penguin Books, New York, 1971.

McCaa, E. (Eagleman), *Mother Earth Spirituality*. HarperCollins, San Francisco, 1990.

Moore, T., *Care of the Soul*. Harper Perennial, New York, 1992.

Ornstein, N., and Sobel, D., *Healthy Pleasures*. Addison-Wesley, Reading, MA, 1990.

Peck, M.S., *The Road Less Traveled*. Touchstone, New York, 1978.

——, *The Different Drum*. Touchstone, New York, 1987.

Pennebaker, J., *Opening Up: The Healing Power of Confiding in Others*. William Morrow & Co., New York, 1990.

Peter, L., and Dana, B., *The Laughter Prescription*. Ballantine, New York, 1982.

Roberts, E., and Amidon, E., *Earth Prayers from Around the World*. Harper, San Francisco, 1991.

Rotter, J., Generalized expectancies for internal versus external control reinforcement. *Psychological Monographs*, 609:80, 1966.

Sams, J., *Earth Medicine*. HarperCollins, San Francisco, 1994.

Sanford, J., *Dreams and Healing*. Paulist Press, New York, 1978.

Schlosser, E., *Fast Food Nation: The Dark Side of the All-American Meal*. Houghton Mifflin, Boston, 2001.

Schaef, A.W., *Co-Dependence: Misunderstood, Mistreated*. Harper and Row, New York, 1986.

Seattle, Chief, A Letter from Chief Seattle, 1855 (from Ed McCaa Eagleman), *Mother Earth Spirituality*. HarperCollins, San Francisco, 1990.

Seaward, B.L., *The Art of Calm: Relaxation through the Five Senses*. Health Communications, Inc., Deerfield Beach, Florida, 1999.

Seaward, B.L., *Health of the Human Spirit: Spiritual Dimensions for Personal Health and Well-Being*. Allyn & Bacon, Inc., Boston, 2000.

Shealy, N., and Myss, C., *The Creation of Health: The Emotional, Psychological and Spiritual Responses That Promote Health and Healing*. Stillpoint Press, Walpole, NH, 1988.

Siegel, B., *Love, Medicine & Miracles*. Perennial, New York, 1987.

——, *Peace, Love, & Healing*. Perennial, New York, 1990.

Simonton, O.C., Simonton, S., and Creighton, J., *Getting Well Again*. Bantam Books, New York, 1978.

Sperry R., The great cerebral commissure. *Scientific American*, 44–52, 1964.

Tannen, D., *That's Not What I Meant! How Conversational Style Makes or Breaks Relationships.* Ballantine Books, New York, 1986.

——, *You Just Don't Understand. Women and Men in Conversation.* Ballantine Books, New York, 1990.

Tietel, M., Wilson, K.A., *Genetically Engineered Food: Changing the Nature of Nature: What You Need to Know to Protect Yourself, Your Family, and Our Planet.* Inner Traditions International, Limited, 2001.

von Oech, R., *A Whack on the Side of the Head.* Warner Books, New York, 1983.

——, *A Kick in the Seat of the Pants.* Perennial Library New York, 1986.

Weisinger, H., *The Anger Workout Book.* Quill Books, Harlinton, TX, 1985.

Yogananda, P., *Inner Reflections.* Self-Realization Fellowship, Los Angeles, CA, 1996.

MORE JOURNAL ENTRIES

ABOUT THE AUTHOR

Brian Luke Seaward is considered a pioneer in the field of health psychology, and he is internationally recognized for his contributions in the area of stress management, human spirituality, and mind–body–spirit healing. The wisdom of Brian Luke Seaward can be found quoted in college lectures, medical seminars, boardroom meetings, church sermons, keynote addresses, and political speeches all over the world. He is respected throughout the international community as an accomplished teacher, consultant, lecturer, author, and mentor. Dr. Seaward has authored over ten books, many published in several languages. He is a faculty member of the University of Colorado at Boulder and the University of Northern Colorado, and his books *Stand Like Mountain, Flow Like Water, Managing Stress, Third Edition*, and *Stressed Is Desserts Spelled Backward* have helped tens of thousands of people overcome personal life crises. When not instructing or presenting stress management programs, Dr. Seaward relaxes back home in the Rocky Mountains of Colorado. He can be reached at www.brianlukeseaward.net.

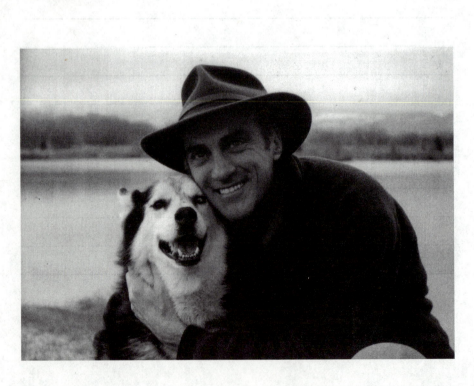